CW00515000

# Will You Read This, Please?

Joanna Cannon graduated from Leicester Medical School and worked as a hospital doctor, before specialising in psychiatry. Her first two novels, *The Trouble with Goats and Sheep* and *Three Things About Elsie*, were both top ten bestsellers and Richard and Judy picks. Her latest novel is *A Tidy Ending*.

# Will You Read This, Please?

EDITED BY

## JOANNA CANNON

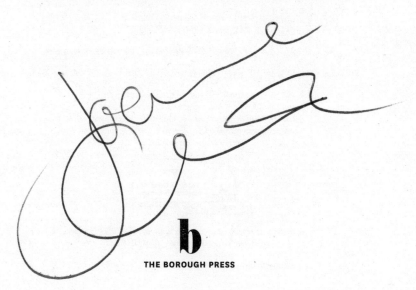

**b**

THE BOROUGH PRESS

The Borough Press
An imprint of HarperCollins*Publishers* Ltd
1 London Bridge Street
London SE1 9GF

www.harpercollins.co.uk

HarperCollins*Publishers*
Macken House, 39/40 Mayor Street Upper,
Dublin 1, D01 C9W8, Ireland

First published by HarperCollins*Publishers* 2023
1

A catalogue record for this book is available from the British Library

HB ISBN: 978-0-00-851997-1
TPB ISBN: 978-0-00-851998-8

Set in Perpetua Std by Palimpsest Book Production Ltd, Falkirk, Stirlingshire

Printed and Bound in the UK using 100% Renewable Electricity at CPI Group (UK) Ltd

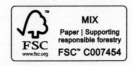

*This book covers a wide range of topics around mental illness, including suicidal ideation, self-harm and eating disorders. A selection of helplines is listed in the back for anyone requiring more information or further support.*

# Contents

# Introduction

Before I began writing novels, I worked as a hospital doctor and my chosen specialty was psychiatry. It was all I ever wanted to do. My uncle had a diagnosis of paranoid schizophrenia and I was fascinated by the many twists and tangles of the human mind, even as a child.

Although I no longer work on the wards, I think of the people I met there every day of my life, and if you read the acknowledgements in any of my books, you will see that I always thank the patients (or service-users, depending on your preference), the *people* I had the privilege to encounter during my career as a medic. Not because I would ever weave them into a novel, but because they changed the way I look at the world. Their courage, wisdom, humour and resilience, often in the presence of huge challenges and social isolation, never failed to amaze me, and even though my life has now taken a different path, their stories will stay with me forever.

I often wondered if there was a way I could bring similar stories to a wider audience, to use the small platform I have built for myself to help others realise the value of lived experience.

Some people who deal with mental illness have the opportunity and ability to write about it, which is amazing, but many do not – and it was those people, those unread stories, I wanted to find. I thought it might be an idea to pair service-users with bestselling authors, to set up a series of collaborations, so the authentic voice of the storyteller was preserved, but it could be shaped and encouraged by someone who wrote stories for a living. Would it work? I had no way of knowing, so one Wednesday lunchtime, I sent out a very tentative tweet asking if anyone thought it was a good idea. I was overwhelmed by the response. Authors, service-users and healthcare professionals all replied with so much support and enthusiasm, and immediately HarperCollins got behind the idea. With the help of the Royal College of Psychiatrists and the power of social media, we asked people with lived experience of mental illness to send in applications. Every application we received was valuable, each one written with huge courage and honesty, but we found our final twelve and matched the story-tellers with eleven talented, compassionate and generous authors (OK, twelve if you count me) who would help these stories to be told. My only conditions were that the stories captured and retained the original voice, and the storytellers were paid the same fee and royalties as the professional authors. I not only wanted them to be heard, I wanted them to be valued. All we needed now was a title, and the title was perhaps the easiest thing of all.

Even when surrounded by the most compassionate and caring staff, someone who is very unwell with mental illness usually doesn't feel heard. *No one listens*, they often say. *No one knows how I feel*. It's also a belief that if we write something down – whether we are unwell or not – we are more likely to be acknowledged, and when I worked as a psychiatrist, I would walk onto the ward each day and find myself approached throughout the morning by a steady trickle of patients with a piece of paper in their hand. They had written down what they wanted to say to me. Long after I'd driven home the previous evening, they had sat on their bed or in the dayroom and found the courage to put their thoughts down onto paper, and as soon as I appeared the next morning they would press that piece of paper into my hands and say, 'Dr Jo, will you read this, please?'

I am so proud of this project. I am in awe of the storytellers for sharing their words and eternally grateful to the authors who helped them to be heard. Most of all I'm proud this book now exists. Because I know if you read this, just like me, your world will be a better place.

Joanna Cannon
November 2022

# Birth Song

## Nicola Knight

### As told to Jenn Ashworth

*Beginnings*

All stories have a beginning. A 'once upon a time'. And now I
am trying to tell mine, I go back to the time after my daughter
was born and try to pinpoint the moment when things started
to go wrong, and I find that I can't. The conditions in the postnatal ward seemed precisely designed to ensure that any moment
of sleep would be interrupted: either by your own crying baby,
or someone else's, or the midwives laughing in the corridor or
someone getting a call on their mobile in the small hours, or
a door slamming, or the endless snoring. Daytimes were difficult
too. We weren't allowed to have the curtains closed around our
beds. The doctors could close them if they wanted privacy when
they pulled up our gowns and inspected our wounds. But we
new mothers weren't allowed to have them closed. Wanting to
sleep or cry without being observed wasn't a good enough
reason, apparently. But wouldn't anyone, in pain, bleeding and
with a body that suddenly felt like it didn't belong to them,
want some privacy?

4

Lots of mothers get emotional after birth, especially after a difficult one. They wrote something to that effect on my notes every day – that I was weepy, emotional, anxious. I want to say now that I was responding, to the trauma of my birth and the total inhumanity of the conditions I was placed in afterwards, in a pretty predictable way. But what happened next was not predictable, was outside the range of what I expected. What anyone expected. Am I saying I started to go mad because the postnatal ward was noisy, and all they cared about was whether I was able to breastfeed my new baby, and I didn't sleep at all for days?

I am, a bit.


*The Krypton Factor*

Time shifts away from me even as I try to catch hold of it. The type of illness I had is not like breaking a leg or having a heart attack where you can point to the calendar and say yes, that's when it happened. I tried with the breastfeeding; I really did. And it hurt me, and the baby lost weight, and I was shamed and embarrassed and pressured and eventually when I decided I wanted to give my baby formula it turned out they'd had bottles of it ready all along. Just sitting there. They brought out this cold-water sterilising bucket you put the tiny pipettes and bottles in to make sure they're clean and safe for a newborn. And it wasn't something I was prepared for – the plan was to breastfeed, and I'd never seen a steriliser before, and for some reason, probably because I was half deranged with tiredness, I just could not get my head around how this thing was supposed to work. My husband – Dan – who had been with me on the ward as much as he was able to, said it was alright, it was fine, that I should stop fiddling with it and leave it alone. It was just a lidded bucket filled with sterilising fluid and all I needed to do was make sure everything in it stayed submerged and we changed the liquid every day. It was not rocket science. But it just didn't *feel* like I was doing it properly. Something was wrong. I kept barking orders at Dan to move it closer, put the lid back on, dip the bottles back under the liquid.

The best way I can describe it is that the steriliser became my adversary. Have you ever seen that old television programme, *The Krypton Factor*? It was on in the late 80s and 90s and the contestants on it would go through all these challenges to test their nerves. There were physical challenges like climbing ropes and scaling nets and crawling on your belly through ditches full of mud. That was the birth, and I'd been through that. Then there were the mental challenges: these impossible puzzles and games involving putting objects together or finding a way through a maze or solving a riddle. It would probably all seem a bit soft now we've got *Big Brother* and *I'm a Celebrity*. But at the time, everyone watched it mainly to see which of the contestants would crack first – because that was the point of the show: to find someone's kryptonite. Apparently, these mental agility tests were designed to be difficult and frustrating – to get some emotional reaction out of the people doing them – but it was actually possible to complete them. Except one time there were two sets of contestants putting together a complicated three-dimensional jigsaw puzzle, racing each other to do it properly, and the production and set people had actually mixed up the pieces by mistake, making each team's puzzle impossible to complete. And apparently these people worked away at it for hours before someone realised something had gone wrong and stepped in. Anyway, that's what it felt like, that impossible steriliser – it was my kryptonite in a game that had been rigged. Because we're all supposed to be superwomen now, aren't we?

Maybe that was the start of it – that urge to get something right, to handle the detail, to be in control. There was so little I'd been able to control – the circumstances of my daughter's birth, the way the medical staff were treating me, the conditions in that bloody awful postnatal ward. I know *everyone* was more or less doing their best. But I know in the midst of that – everyone doing what they thought they needed to do – who I was and what I needed was kind of lost. I was lost.


## The Right Words

Maybe talking about a steriliser is a strange way to start this story. But it's actually kind of hard to talk about at all – what happened, what it felt like, what it meant to me at the time and what it means now. I don't say the word 'psychosis' out loud too often. I'm a writer – considering words and language is what I do all the time. Always have. I love to read, love to be swimming in words and stories. I'm writing a novel about this time and one day I'm going to be able to get the whole experience onto paper and say something important about the way the NHS cares for babies at the expense of pregnant women and new mothers, and how we talk or don't talk about mental health; about fear and politeness getting in the way of connecting with someone who has lost their own connection to the real world.

But first I have to get a grip on the words. If I don't say 'psychosis', what do I say? 'The time I was ill'? or 'The time after my daughter was born'? or 'That time I went mad / lost my mind / went loopy'? On the online message boards, people hardly ever type it out. They write 'PPP' or PNP' and let the initials do the work. Dan and I skate past it sometimes: as painful for him, in ways that I might never understand, as it was for me. 'That time when you were ill,' he says. Or 'You know, when Grace was first born,' and nods meaningfully. And we do that partly because it still hurts, and partly because *psychosis* is sometimes a word too scary to say out loud.

It's scary for other people too. There are statistics you can find online about how many women kill themselves in the first year after having a baby, how many are hospitalised, how many kill their own babies. There are lists of symptoms and signs – usually aimed at the partner or caregiver, because the assumption is that when you're that far gone, you yourself are the least likely person to know that you are sick.

I searched for these lists of symptoms sometimes, even in the early days while it was all happening. I was sick, but I wasn't stupid. I made notes on my mobile phone, trying to capture everything – not only about how often the baby was feeding but about my moods, about the strange things I was thinking and worrying about. I was keeping tabs on the wound from my C-section. Keeping it clean and making sure it was healing properly. But somehow, quite quickly, that checking went into overdrive and I was convinced that the wound had started to rot, that it smelled bad, that my body was falling to bits. I kept careful records of this. I noted the way the wound and my feelings about it changed. I asked Google a million different questions. I knew something was going wrong, and once I explained to a midwife what was happening. I'd looked up 'postpartum psychosis' on my phone and I showed her the article. I told her I thought that was what I had. Was having.

'Oh, I heard of a woman who had that,' she said breezily. 'She took off all her clothes and ran down the street, apparently.' She laughed, and we both imagined her, that woman – stripped naked and running down the road. I worried about her feet – her bare feet. This woman, running away from her baby, from her life, from everything. And towards what? And the idea of this woman and what her illness had driven her to was funny, apparently. At least it was to the midwife I tried to speak to.

'Now you're not about to do anything like that, are you, dear?' she said comfortably, knowledgeably. I looked down at myself. I was holding a cup of tea I couldn't remember making and I was, in fact, wearing something – a dressing gown. I had slippers and socks on my feet. So, I must have been all right. Right?

*Certainty*

The birth itself was horrendous. The baby was too big, too late, too high up, not far down enough. The labour was late, absent, too slow. There were examinations and inductions and endless, endless waiting while nothing happened. It hurt. It was humiliating. It was not what I'd planned or hoped for – and I know these things aren't under your control and I know that sometimes nature needs help. But I felt, in the end, like a piece of meat being inspected, wheeled around, poked and prodded at, and found wanting. There was 'failure to progress', which is a phrase you're not supposed to take personally but how can you not? I had one job in there, which was to get the baby out. And I was medically diagnosed as a failure. When the baby's heart rate began to increase, the labour ended in a C-section which itself ended with a surgeon and a couple of nurses pushing down hard at the top of my bump and me being dragged halfway down the table. They say you're not supposed to feel it because of the anaesthetic, but you do, and it isn't exactly pain but your body knows it is being attacked and the part of you that knows is in terror. And then the baby. We hadn't asked the sonographer to tell us if we were having a boy or a girl. But I knew. I just knew. And when they finally got her out and held her up, wailing, I could see she was a girl just as I'd expected and the sheer joy of her being born and that trust I felt in myself, my own body, my knowledge of it and her safe arrival burst out of me like a song and lit up the room like sunshine. Afterwards, the surgeon said, 'You'd never have got that baby out on your own,' and she was big – gloriously so – and him saying that made me feel vindicated.

I'm calling my daughter Grace, for this story. It isn't her real name, but it means love – a kind of excessive love that you don't deserve and that it isn't possible to earn, but that you get anyway. A kind of love you can be certain of. And I was certain of her – and I clung to that, through all the days that followed and into now.

### Heavenly Light

Other moments, I'm less sure of and perhaps I won't ever be. And that's hard to accept.

Early on, just a few days after we'd come home from hospital my family came to see me. They came a lot in the early days – at first to see the new baby, then as it became clear that I wasn't sleeping and something was wrong, to help Dan look after her and me. My sister came and brought her own baby. We were in my bedroom and my niece was sitting on the bed on top of the duvet, my sister hovering nearby to make sure she was safe. She looked so big compared to Grace. The bedroom had turned into a chaotic nest, full of the detritus of early motherhood. The curtains were half drawn the way they are when you're sleeping at odd hours, or not sleeping, and your sense of whether it is four in the afternoon or four in the morning is becoming unstitched from itself. What I mean to say is, the light was pouring through the half-drawn curtain, casting the corners of the room into shadow. The light fell directly onto the bed and while my sister was speaking to me and as I was searching the top of the nightstand for something, I turned and saw that sunshine cover my niece and I saw how beautiful and good she was. She was glowing.

Lots of people feel like that about their own children and the children in their family – that they're special in some way. And all babies are beautiful and gifts from God: every birth is a song of praise, in its way. But there was something else – some quality of the light that made it seem that the sun itself was searching out my niece and wanted to touch her, wanted to be near her. My thoughts ran on like this and it didn't feel like a mad thing to be thinking; it felt like love. Perhaps it was. Should I have noticed that? Should I have said something to my sister – something about the way the light flooded through the curtains and touched her daughter's skin and illuminated the translucent fluff of her hair and made it look not only like she had a halo, but like her whole body was glowing – as if the light wasn't really coming in from the outside and hitting her (I could see that it was) but that the truth of the matter was the light was coming out of her – that this baby sitting on my bed was making the light? Should my sister have noticed me staring and said something?


*The Case of the Disappearing Cats*

There were other 'visual disturbances', as the textbooks describe it. We have cats – a pair of cats – and before we had the real

11

baby, they were my babies (they still are). These cats were loved and pampered and properly looked after but one morning, in the week or so after I'd come back from the hospital, I saw them curled up on their bed and had the thought that they looked a bit skinny. This might have been the light or the way they were lying. Maybe they'd gone off their food during the time I was in hospital and had lost a little weight. But as I listened to that thought – *they're looking a bit thin* – it seemed to me that they were emaciated, lying there too weak to move.

I called the vet and made an appointment for them both to be checked over. That is a sane thing to do: it's what any responsible cat owner would do. Then I looked at them again and decided no, I'd been seeing things, they were fine. So I cancelled the appointment. But in the next moment, they looked almost skeletal, and I worried they'd been eaten away by something – that they had worms or parasites or some fast-acting cancer. And what would people think if I devoted all my time and energies to the new baby and didn't bother getting medical help for them? Dan assured me they were fine. But did I listen? No. So I called the vet again and remade the appointments. Then I worried that when the vet saw the state of them, she would call the RSPCA and we'd get into trouble. So I cancelled the appointments again. It went on like that, all afternoon. The cats carried on lying where they were, sunning themselves, sleeping and licking their paws. In the end, I paid a fortune for an out-of-hours appointment and my friends – not cat people at all – took them in and they were fine.

I wonder if the impression I had that the cats were starving was really to do with my guilt about them taking a bit of a back seat to all the drama and chaos of a new baby in the house. Or if it was more of the same worry and sense of loss of control that I'd felt when faced with that steriliser, or the task of understanding how much milk the baby had drunk at any particular feed. It is tempting to try and read these delusions and impressions as if they hold the key to what was happening in my head and heart and to my life at that time. But perhaps it was just chemicals, and my brain going wrong, and the attempt to make some meaning of it is a waste of time.

*Drug Resistant*

Around this time a GP came to the house to see me. I tried to explain what had been going on. It's strange to say I have a happy memory of this man, despite how distressed I was at that time and how it's still so painful to think about, but I do. It's not that other people didn't care – Dan was swinging between being worried sick and assuming that the racing thoughts, the manic pacing, the panic, the worry, the irritability, was just what new mothers were like. All the parenting books say that, don't they? That a husband can expect his wife to be a little erratic in the days and weeks after birth. A little tearful and oversensitive. My family were there too, helping with the practical things, and when I ran around the house wearing only a towel and insisted that my clothes were nowhere to be found, were lost, had gone missing, they tried to get me tucked into bed with a cup of tea: everyone thought that all I needed was sleep.

Then this doctor arrived – an older male GP who I didn't think would understand, and who asked me some questions. I can't remember what I said, but I remember him nodding and me feeling that yes, finally someone got it – something serious was happening with me.

'Your thoughts are racing, you can't catch up with yourself, is that right?' he said, and there was such a kindness in his tone.

13

(Now I'm remembering this, I'm wondering if that was part of the illness too, that powerful sense of understanding – almost love – I felt from him, and my gratitude for it. How would I ever know?) He went outside into the street and made a call on his mobile, then he came back with a prescription for some heavy-duty sleeping pills.

'These are going to put you to sleep,' he said, handing them over, 'and a full night's sleep will make everything feel a lot better. Will you take them for me?' He checked with Dan that he was OK to take care of the baby, then gave me the prescription. And he didn't imply that the problem was just a lack of sleep and nothing more, only that getting a full night was going to help me. So I took the pills, went to bed and dozed for an hour then sat up all night, my mind vibrating and my eyeballs shaking in their sockets. I was totally out of it, but still awake. That was the night I saw the grasshoppers. They were lurid neon green, impossible to ignore – crawling up and down my arms. They were so real. I picked one off my skin and squashed it between my fingers. I felt it burst. I didn't imagine I felt it or dream I felt it. I *felt it* burst. Then they all vanished, leaving me frozen with horror.

*Crisis*

When everything came to a head, it wasn't actually because I was losing my mind – though I was. It was because I thought I was having a heart attack. I was lying in my bed with my entire body shaking. It felt like my heart was going to break its way through my ribs. I'd become convinced I could control my own breathing and heart rate. That I could kill myself if I wanted to, with my own mind. Then I started to panic, my vision started to blur and I began to lose control of my thoughts all together.

14

Perhaps the paramedics didn't really think it was my heart, but they had to be careful with women who've had C-sections because of blood clots in the lungs and other complications, and they could see that I was unravelling and thought this was a good enough way to get me into hospital.

I was lying in bed when they arrived and I was so confused, hearing the swiping, chopping sounds of a helicopter overhead, those steady deep notes like a percussion I couldn't only hear, but could feel, echoing and vibrating around my body. *They've sent an air ambulance*, I thought, my head on the pillow. I remembered that Prince William flew helicopters. Was that his job? Did he fly down and pick up people who were having heart attacks or panic attacks or whose brains were exploding through lack of sleep? My head on the pillow, my heart racing, my skin tacky with sweat, I imagined Prince William in his helicopter, hovering over the house, and a paramedic dangling on a rope coming down to rescue me from the dark, narrow place I was trapped in – as if I had fallen down a well. Of course, there was no helicopter, just an ordinary run-of-the-mill ambulance, and I think that sound I was hearing – that whooshing, flickering, *thwock-thwock-thwock* sound, so loud it was shaking the house and must have been coming from outside – was the sound of my own heart beating in panic, the blood thundering in my ears.

*God*

And that's another thing. My whole life, when things have been frightening or confusing, I have turned to God as a refuge. My church community. The Bible. We all need something to trust. Something to rely on when everything else falls apart. And I knew – and have based my life around this certain faith – that

I was cared for by God and that God would never abandon me. At the worst point, when I couldn't remember anything from the Bible, the names of any of the friends who would have supported me, and when I couldn't even pray, I went to the mirror and looked into my own eyes. I don't know what I was looking for. My soul, maybe. The part of me – that divine light or spark – that is of God. That shining goodness we see in babies and young children that glows right out of them and then fades a bit as we get older and get dirtied up by the rough and tumble of the fallen world. I looked for that. And I didn't recognise the person I saw in the mirror. The person staring back at me had black eyes, pinprick pupils, wild hair. Looked otherworldly, somehow. Dark. I could remember the name of Jesus, and I said it out loud a few times, instead of a prayer, desperately hoping to be heard, knowing that I sounded very, very far gone, and not knowing how to come back.

But when you're standing in a hospital convinced that you could stop your heart with the power of your own mind and you really want to be taken seriously, you know you can't mention God. There is a difference between having faith and being ill, but there's something in our culture that often assumes a person with a strong faith in God is someone to avoid, someone to be afraid of. This is a difficult thing to admit to, but I kept my mouth shut about God while I was in hospital because I was scared they'd take Grace away from me.

## Hospital

It felt important, once the paramedics delivered me to hospital, to make sure they knew I wasn't mental. I know that kind of language offends some people. But this is my story. My words.

16

I wanted them to know I wasn't a 'problem person': I was a professional woman, even though I looked wild at that time – dressing gown a bit tatty and my hair all over the place. I looked like someone who was falling apart, but it became important to me that they saw me as an adult and as a person worthy of respect. So I answered their questions as carefully as I could. And I wasn't entirely honest about how I'd been feeling. You always know, you see, no matter how far you've gone, that they can take the baby away from you. At any given moment, someone can make that call. But the way I presented myself must have worked: they sent me home, and it wasn't until I called the crisis team myself a few days later that I started to get some of the help that I needed.

The members of that team came with care and love and they listened in a way that no one else had and they treated me like a human being, not something to be afraid of. It was only much later that I discovered how close I had come to being sectioned, separated from Grace just as I always feared and sent across the country for treatment. But no, they elected to treat me at home, the local perinatal mental health team visiting me – us – regularly, for over a year, with psychologist appointments and more sleeping pills and time to talk whenever I needed it. And although it was really only the beginning of my recovery, it was a beginning. It was as if someone – not Prince William this time, but some everyday, heroic nurses – had reached down to pull me out of a deep, deep well, just when I thought all hope was lost.


*In Retrospect*

So now I'm better. That's one way of ending this story, I suppose. I was rescued. And that would be part of the truth: I'm no longer in that dark place, but I exist on the edge of that deep hole now, and live my life precariously, knowing it is there. It's difficult to explain.

So – I work with horses. Not directly, but I do communications for a charity that works with horses. And while I was sick, before that kind GP came to see me and the paramedics came and took me to hospital, I was convinced that I was seeing worms – the type that sick horses get if they're not looked after properly – in the carpet on the upstairs landing. A nasty little clump of worms just lying there, wriggling. In the actual carpet. And I reacted the way most sane people would react if they had a newborn in the house and parasites in the soft furnishings: I wanted them out, gone, right away. My thoughts were a swarm and all I could think about was cleaning – cleaning for hours, scrubbing everything, and buying things on the internet to prevent rats, to keep the house clean and safe, to control the worms that were infesting the place.

It's obviously not something I bring up in day-to-day conversation. Nobody who was around at that time – my husband, my parents, who were coming every day to help – is likely to say, 'Hey, Nicola, remember that time you thought you saw worms in the carpet, ha ha,' are they? So it's a little detail that's just been lying there, un-thought about, for years. Like a pair of jeans you forgot about, then find one day tucked into the back of a drawer when you were looking for something else. So the difficult thing isn't that I saw worms in the carpet when I was sick, but instead that it's only recently – like, really, really recently – when I pulled those jeans out of the drawer and held them up to the light, it was only then that I decided no, they weren't worms after all. That was a hallucination. Probably.

It's good, I suppose. Recalibrating my past and getting the real world and the imagined world in the right place. But it makes the future scary, too. Not because I think I might get sick again – I try not to think about that – but because there will be more details I have to reorganise like this. More memories that turn out to be delusions, more events or ideas that I have to move from the 'this happened' to the 'this probably didn't happen' box. The past, for me, is an unstable, untrustworthy thing, and that is an important part of what 'recovery' looks like.

## Garden Centre

I still struggle with anger sometimes. Don't get me wrong – deep down I know it wasn't anyone's fault, exactly, that I was sick. Yes, I could have been cared for better – more humanely. And yes, the conditions in the postnatal ward afterwards could have been set up so that women like me, women who'd had major surgery and needed to recover physically and emotionally – could have sleep. Maybe there was a different kind of cruelty in the old days of swiping the babies away from their mothers and lining them up in cots in nurseries to be fed every four hours and not before. But there's a cruelty in the way we do things now, turning women into vessels and milk machines and prioritising what the baby needs at all costs. Can't women matter too?

I still can't be without my sleep – a late night can trigger insomnia, and if there's any sense that sleep will be prevented or interrupted, I can panic and get angry. A few nights ago, my friend wanted me to stay up late and watch *Eurovision* with her – she was insisting, playfully, and pretending not to take no for an answer and I lost it a little bit with her in the end. I could tell she didn't get it. Not really. And you can explain as much as you like – *if I don't sleep I might go mad* – but how can you really explain that to anyone in a way that they totally and completely understand? Not mad as in being a bit irritable and weepy and needing a coffee and a lot of sugar in the late afternoon type of mad. Not mad as in forgetful or dozy or nodding off in front of the telly in the early evening sort of mad. But seeing things that aren't there sort of mad. You can't explain that to anyone, so it sets up a distance between people who you've previously been really close to; you've had this experience that has marked and changed you forever, and they haven't. That's another part of what recovery looks like: once you know that well is there, and it is possible to fall down it, you have to be vigilant that you don't. Things that were once easy are less easy now, and I'm angry about that too.

I was talking about it with my mum a few weeks ago. We were in a café at a garden centre, and Grace was playing with some toys on the floor by the window. The window was one of those floor-to-ceiling ones and through it I could see the counters and tables full of flowers – the pinks and whites and yellows – and sense that living, earthy, warm smell they have in garden centres. It was a normal day – the way normal always feels like a special treat now, after lockdown, after what happened. And I was watching Grace over by the window and I guess a cloud shifted and the sun came out and suddenly she was sitting as if in a spotlight and I had these two thoughts at the same time – the first was how lovely she is, and how glad I am to have her, and of course how having a healthy baby counts for a lot – it always did. It took me back to that moment I first saw her – that utter joy not only in her, but in my own mind, in knowing I'd been right and she'd been a girl all along. My daughter. And there was the second thought, seeing her sitting in the sunlight like that, the glow of it touching her hair and the back of her

20

neck and the shoulder of her coat – nothing special, just this tatty anorak we put her in for the park – that she was glowing. *She's glowing*, I thought; then I got scared. Is that an all right thought to think? Is that me going mad again? Do other people think like that? All of this, crashing about inside me in the time it took me to pour some milk into my tea and lift my mug. And my mum, who has often asked if she let me down by not spotting what was wrong with me sooner, noticed that something was happening in that moment.

'Are you OK?' she asked.

And the real answer is, I don't know. I don't know if I am OK. I can't always tell. And just because I am OK now, in this minute, doesn't mean that I can feel certain I will be OK in the next minute, or the one after that. Mum stirred her tea and buttered a scone and waited for me to answer.

*I never knew*, I wanted to tell her – I never knew it was possible to seem OK to the outside world, but inside my mind could turn into a kind of chaos that even years later I would struggle to understand. I couldn't say any of this. I never say any of this. She followed my gaze to where Grace was sitting in the light, still playing with those toys that were too young for her. It was a wooden ark, and some of the animals had lost their pairs so she had Mrs Giraffe lined up with Mr Elephant and Mrs Swan with Mr Pig. The light spilled down over everything; my mother waited, and still I didn't answer.

'I heard voices after you were born,' she said lightly, as if it didn't matter. She was looking away from me as if she didn't want to see my reaction, and we were both looking towards Grace, sitting there in the light in front of the glass windows, the brightness of the flowers behind her as vivid as a song.

# Do No Harm

## Marie

### As told to Benjamin Johncock

1.

*It's early January, late evening, and I'm terrified by the thoughts in my head. Graphic thoughts of violence towards those closest to me. I can't make them stop. I feel like I'm being tortured by my own mind. It's horrific. It's 2014, I'm living with my parents, but tonight I'm home alone. What's happening to me? I decide to get rid of all the knives — and any other dangerous implements — from the house. I don't want them here. I find an old hold-all and carry it through to the kitchen. I open the cutlery drawer and start filling the bag with anything sharp. I take the poker from the fireplace too. I zip up the bag, put on my coat, step out into the cold night. This is my hometown. This is where I grew up. I walk down to the bay area. It's not far from the house. The sea is a fury and the wind bites at my face. I unzip the hold-all and dump everything into the black water. The rocks are wet and I slip over, gashing my knee. It's very dark. I can't see what I'm doing. My knee hurts. I manage to stand up and get myself off the rocks. I limp home, bloody and tired. I'm a shy, bookish, thirty-seven-year-old woman who feels bad if they ever have to flush a spider down the drain. How have*

*I become someone so terrified of harming those I love that I've dumped a bag full of knives into the North Sea at night like a gangster disposing of evidence? Things have gone too far. I need help. I don't yet know that I'm suffering from a common subset of obsessive–compulsive disorder, called Harm OCD. With no outwardly observable compulsions, it's often called Pure OCD, or Pure O. I won't have this diagnosis – or the tools to help me get better – for a long time.*

## 2.

On the easternmost point of mainland Scotland, an hour's drive north of Aberdeen, there's a small but busy fishing port with majestic views over the sea. Reddish-brown ashlar stone buildings line the long streets that fan out from the harbour; their distinctive granite mined from local quarries a long time ago. The town has pockets of deprivation and pockets of wealth, like so many on the coast. It even gets a mention in Jules Verne's 1864 novel, *Journey to the Centre of the Earth*. I've lived here all my life. My childhood dream was to be a writer. I went to the local comprehensive school, then studied English Literature at Aberdeen University. The remains of Slaine Castle nearby are thought to have inspired Bram Stoker when he was writing *Dracula*. He'd have month-long writing holidays in the area. I've always had a strong imagination too. I think the building blocks for my OCD were probably there from an early stage in life. I was sensitive and prone to rumination, and I've always struggled with uncertainty. I've always erred on the side of caution and safety, often overestimating risk. And I think that my strong imaginative capacity has been a double-edged sword in my life. Where Bram Stoker imagined Dracula, my mind would go on to imagine far more frightening things.

3.

In 2010, when I was thirty-two years old, I started to have serious panic attacks. I thought something dreadful was going to happen to me – that I was going to have a heart attack, or collapse, or something else equally bad. The panic attacks quickly snowballed into agoraphobia and my world suddenly became very constricted – even going around the block was a real struggle. I was completely blindsided. It was incredibly hard to access any kind of therapy in 2010 – and it was an entire year before I was offered anything on the NHS. I had a short course of outpatient therapy with a clinical psychologist but, ironically, as an outpatient, I was required to travel to Aberdeen. It sounds like something from *Catch-22*: if you suffer from agoraphobia, you can't get any treatment unless you leave the house and travel a considerable distance. Once I'd started, I was able to go out a bit more, although I wasn't doing anything beyond strict routines. For two or three years, my world was very circumscribed. I was having trouble finding a job, getting established, settling into something. I was spending a good deal of time on my own at home, reading newspapers, watching TV. I was in a vulnerable state. Things were about to get much worse. I was reading news reports of the Lee Rigby murder trial that took place at the end of 2013. In the press coverage, I learned that the murderers, Michael Adebolajo and Michael Adebowale, had bought kitchen knives in a high-street store: it was the ostensible trigger of my OCD.

4.

*The idea of* harm *has taken over my brain. I'm in the supermarket. I steer well clear of the aisle with the kitchen knives. It soon starts spreading like a fungus to every part of my life. Scissors are terrifying — as is the fire poker. I banish steak knives and bread knives to the boot of the car. Every morning I wake up in a state of dread. It's not the anxiety I'm familiar with from the panic attacks though — this is something different. I try to avoid any possible trigger. I stop being able to do simple things, like look in the cutlery drawer in the kitchen. I stop functioning. I'm constantly asking myself,* what does this mean?

## 5.

I didn't know it at the time, but my brain was incorrectly interpreting my thoughts as a signal; a warning – of danger. I'd also learn that my constant questioning of *why* I was having these thoughts was inadvertently attributing importance to them, making them even stickier. I was stuck in a hellish parallel universe.

## 6.

*It's the day after I carried the hold-all down to the cold, dark water of the North Sea. I phone up an NHS mental health helpline and explain everything to them. The horror scenarios going through my mind are just too much. I'm being bombarded, like junk email, and I can't get them to stop. With the panic attacks, I was scared for myself, but now, I'm scared for* other *people. What do these violent thoughts mean? Where are they coming from? Do I need to be locked up? Am I losing my mind? The woman I speak to recognises that I'm not well. She tells me to hang up and make an appointment to see someone. I go to my GP, who has been my family doctor for as long as I can remember. I know I have to be upfront and honest, but as I talk, I see her professional demeanour slip — she looks taken aback; a little disturbed — I can see it in her face. She tells me that I need to see a mental health specialist; it's obviously something that needs looking into. I'm going to be fast-tracked on the NHS but there's no telling when I'll get seen. In the meantime, she books me a private appointment. I leave the surgery. I'm very scared. I'm clearly psychotic.*

## 7.

My GP didn't say anything about OCD. I don't think she recognised it; I had to piece the puzzle together on my own. I looked online. I'd heard of OCD before, but the Disneyfied version of it; the version you get in popular culture, where it's just about checking things like light switches, and obsessive hand-washing. I found some forums on the internet where people were talking about it; I read about mothers with postpartum OCD, terrified of harming their babies. I didn't have a child, but I could relate to them. People talked about bizarre urges they'd get, like driving off the road when they were in the car, or deliberately smashing into a wall. That there was this community of other people online with similar experiences to mine was both helpful and comforting. The shame factor surrounding Harm OCD meant that I didn't feel able to broach the issue with family and friends.

## 8.

*My GP puts me on a selective serotonin reuptake inhibitor — or SSRI, for short; an antidepressant. They're used to treat a range of psychological conditions, including anxiety disorders. But they're not working* for me. I see a second doctor, at the same practice. I give him the whole story again, expecting him to be horrified. But he's not as concerned as my original GP. He's much more blasé. It's reassuring. I ask him if he thinks I'm psychotic. He gives a small laugh, says kindly, 'Oh no, I don't think you're psychotic.' He doesn't have answers but his demeanour tells me that he's not disturbed by what I'm saying. He suggests switching my current SSRI to another that he's had more success with: sertraline.

## 9.

Reading the enormous fold-out instruction leaflet of any SSRI is always a slightly terrifying and depressing experience, not least because it states that you may experience an intensifying of symptoms before they work. I read through them and wondered how things could possibly get any more intense for me. But that's exactly what did happen. I wasn't sleeping at all – not a wink. My brain was in overdrive. I was just not functioning. This went on for nearly two weeks, until I finally told my parents, *I need to go into a hospital.*

## 10.

Dad drives me back to the surgery. I've managed to get one of those last-minute appointments at the end of the day. It's half-seven, dark outside; cold. The doctor just wants to go home. He's not particularly nice. I tell him, I feel like I'm going out of my mind. He asks questions – questions I know he has to ask – but there's no empathy, no care. Would you harm yourself? How would you go about it? Those questions. He says he can get me admitted tonight, if I want. The Royal Cornhill

27

is a psychiatric hospital in Aberdeen wedged between Westburn skatepark and Berryden Retail Park. It's Friday night. Aberdeen is an hour by car. I'd have to be assessed when I got there, and he tells me this could take several hours. I ask if he can arrange it for the morning, as I'd like my dad to come with me for support – going into a psychiatric hospital is quite a big deal if you've never been an inpatient before, and my dad's been working hard all day. I don't want him sitting up into the wee hours waiting for me to be assessed and then driving back home. The doctor says, 'Well, just go in by yourself! Don't bother your dad.' It's unbelievable.

## 11.

It was a very worrying time for my parents. They had tried to jolly me out of it at the start, but as it progressed, they realised it wasn't something I could just shake off. They soon started to notice things – things like, *where are all the knives?* Things were disappearing around the house. What happened to the scissors? So they talked to me, asked me what was going on. Mum found it strange and unsettling, I think because she had just had surgery and was feeling a bit vulnerable herself. It was hard for her to listen to. Dad was more matter-of-fact. He thought it was probably just stress that had taken some weird form – nothing to really worry about. He didn't want me being admitted. He thought it would make things worse, as he knows what a sensitive person I am. I don't think he really understood at the time what was going on internally for me. Nobody wants to be in a psychiatric hospital. I just wanted to be in an environment where I couldn't possibly harm anyone. I wanted peace after so many sleepless nights, waking up to horrible thoughts that I couldn't escape from.

## 12.

*Dad takes me down to the Royal Cornhill on Saturday morning. I'm assessed by a young psychiatrist, who doesn't think I need to be sectioned. He asks if I want to be admitted. I have my bag with me, packed for this eventuality, but I know I'm on my own in this decision. I say yes, please. And that's it. I say goodbye to my dad, and the young psychiatrist takes me up to the ward where I'll end up spending the next four months.*

## 13.

The wards were all named after Scottish castles. I was in *Glamis*, the childhood home of the Queen Mother. I've never been to Glamis Castle; I doubt I'll ever want to now. The ward had a dining area and a small kitchen, as well as a lounge that I never found very inviting. The main hospital entrance was modern, with artwork hanging on the walls, but the wards were drab and dingy. As a physical environment, it had a depressing effect. I had my own room for the first six weeks or so because I really didn't want to be around other people. After that, I was in a single-sex dormitory with about four or five other women. The morning after my admission, I was seen by a really lovely psychiatrist who was just about to retire. He was just filling in that weekend. And he gave me my OCD diagnosis. He was so laid-back about it: *Don't worry. I've seen this all before. You're not going to harm anyone. There's nothing new under the sun. You're not psychotic. It's OCD.* It was so immensely reassuring! He told me that I had a hard road ahead. There were no quick fixes with OCD.

## 14.

*I keep my diagnosis from the other patients; I dread being labelled as dangerous. Even though I'm in a controlled environment now, I can still see the potential for harm everywhere. What's to stop me stabbing another patient in the eye with the fork in my hand? Night time in the dormitory is torture: people are asleep and defenceless in their beds. I'm bombarded with violent, intrusive thoughts that leave me in a near-permanent state of high anxiety. The woman in the bed next to me is snoring loudly again.* I lie awake thinking, what if I go berserk and strangle her? *My other bedside neighbour is an older woman who enjoys knitting. When her partner comes to visit, she goes off to the visiting area to see him, leaving her knitting needles in her bedside cabinet. She doesn't know that I have Harm OCD. She doesn't know that I'm plagued with thoughts of skewering her with those knitting needles in a fit of rage. I find it so stressful that I ask one of the nurses to take the needles away until she returns. Everyone on the ward has different problems – unless you choose to tell others, they don't know.*

## 15.

I had twice-weekly sessions with the ward psychiatrist, agonising over how much I could really tell them, as well as a weekly exposure session with another member of staff, and daily chats with the psychiatric nurses. My first regular psychiatrist was very empathetic, although unrealistic about the severity of my condition. She thought I'd be able to go home in the middle of February, after only a month. She wanted to schedule a meeting for my discharge. There was no way I was going to be ready to go home in just four weeks. Meanwhile, I still wasn't having any luck with the SSRI that I was taking. It just wasn't gelling with my brain chemistry. I felt really worked up on it. Finally, one of the psychiatrists did a bit of research on another class of drugs, called tricyclics, and we had a breakthrough. He prescribed clomipramine, and slowly this medication began to work for me. The terrifying scenarios started to fade in their intensity.

16.

*Mum and Dad bring me in books when they visit, as well as notepads and pens so I can do creative writing — things they think I can immerse myself in — but my bandwidth is so contracted that reading is so strained, and the thoughts are always there. You can't read and not have the thoughts — it just doesn't work like that.*

17.

As with most disorders, OCD has various sub-types. There was a young woman on my ward who had what you might call classic OCD — that is, the highly visible kind that involved repeatedly touching things and rearranging objects. She would hold up people who were trying to get into the dining room by continually touching the door, and she flushed the toilet numerous times during the night. At the time, with my skewed thinking, I perceived her as having a more legitimate form of the illness — one that got her more attention from the staff. I sometimes felt as though my suffering was going unnoticed because my OCD was invisible. No one made jokes about it in popular culture. It felt like I wasn't receiving the same level of support. Mental illness makes you so self-absorbed. The psychiatric nurses had a hell of a job to do — and they were on their feet all day, working twelve-hour shifts. They were very good, all of them, but it was always a case of trying to attract their attention as they went from patient to patient, checking in on everybody. The state I was in, I suppose I was jealous of the more visible issues that some patients presented with. I felt like I couldn't just go up to one of the nurses and say, I'm having a thought about randomly stabbing someone. It didn't feel like the same kind of thing. My feelings towards this woman only thawed when I found myself alone in the ward kitchen with her. She was making a cup of tea and she suddenly broke down in tears. She said, 'I don't want to be here – this illness has taken me away from my family.' At that moment I realised making category distinctions between her OCD and my OCD was invidious. Both of us were suffering equally, and in fundamentally similar ways. There were probably other kinds of OCD affecting those around me that I didn't even recognise. I shared a dormitory with an elderly lady in her late sixties. We enjoyed daily conversations but neither of us divulged our conditions to each other. I remember that quite often, several hours after we'd had a conversation, she'd come up to me in the ward and ask, 'I haven't offended you, have I?' At the time I just thought it was an amusing aspect of her personality that I occasionally found annoying. I even wondered if she might have dementia. Looking back now, though, I think this could have been a manifestation of OCD that I simply wasn't familiar with.

18.

I had a couple of hour-long sessions with a clinical psychologist as well as the psychiatrists. I was encouraged to stop trying to find an underlying meaning for the thoughts that I was being plagued by and try to focus more on the meta-cognitive side of things. It was about being able to just accept the thoughts and detach yourself from them; not see them as being bound up with your identity. I also learned about the thought–action fusion, which was such an ingrained feature of my thinking, where you believe that simply thinking about an action is the same as actually carrying out that action. It's a sort of cognitive error. The psychologist watched me hold a serrated knife in my hand and lived to tell the tale. She also encouraged me to try and think of my OCD not as a fundamental flaw, but more as a kind of brain hiccup (distressing, but harmless). I was only able to get two of these hour-long sessions with the clinical psychologist in my whole four-month stay as an inpatient; a very clear reflection of staffing issues and the strain on the service.

## 19.

*I force myself to buy a newspaper every day and read it, even though I know it will contain articles about violence. A lot of the time, though, I cheat and only skim the headlines, because of what triggered my OCD in the first place. I don't want any more violent ideas or images implanted in my brain, but I do want to stay connected to the real world. The occupational therapist takes me out into the centre of Aberdeen, on public transport, to be around people again and avoid becoming institutionalised. It's pretty disconcerting. I become hyper-aware of things. I always worry in case I do or say something that makes people know I'm a mental hospital patient. And I try to spend as much time out of the ward as possible. The hospital grounds are landscaped and mildly uplifting, so I begin doing circuit walks as winter slowly starts to creep towards spring.*

20.

And then, four months after my admission, I was discharged. I still felt in a highly vulnerable state. I still didn't trust myself. To be at home again and told to get on with it; to live with these objects that had caused me so much distress before – but that are part of everyday life – was very difficult. It took time. I had monthly catch-ups at my GP surgery with my psychiatrist to review medication, and fortnightly sessions as an outpatient with a clinical psychologist at the hospital and with a community psychiatric nurse at home. One of the things I had to do at home was prepare dinner in front of my mum. And that was when I went back to the cutlery drawer and started to reacquaint myself with its contents. I think I did this with them both watching on at least half a dozen occasions. Six months after I was discharged, I was still far from being 'cured' – there remained recurrent, troubling thoughts, and I still had a phobia of sharp objects – but with most mental illnesses like OCD, I don't think there's a *Eureka!* moment when you can just move on. My daily life was still a struggle for many, many months. My therapy sessions gave me a much better understanding of OCD, though – and equipped me with tools and strategies to help. I think it was a good year and a half before I began to feel even semi-normal again.


21.

I've now got a job in the cultural sector doing work that I love. Clomipramine has been a godsend. I wish I'd taken antidepressants sooner; they might have saved me years of lost productivity. I've been taking them for almost eight years and

I'm now on the lowest dose, ready to be weaned off. They've got side effects – all medicines do – but they've worked for me. I never like to think that all this couldn't come back sometime, but I know what OCD is now – what it *really* is, even if it took on another form and presented as a different subset.


22.

There's not enough awareness of the spectrum of mental health conditions at the primary care level – and I think that's a real problem. GPs just aren't equipped to deal with people in crisis. I don't think they know what to do. There was no awareness of the extreme distress I was in. And no one made contact out of hours to check up on me, or ask how I was coping. You see a GP for your appointment – and that's it. In a mental health context, it's not enough. They didn't even recommend help plans for me to go on, or people to speak to – I had to do my own internet research. There should be *far* more prevention going on within the primary care setting, not just prescribing SSRIs and telling people to battle it out. I do think, though, that there's been much more awareness, generally, around mental health over the last few years. It's definitely percolated into the culture more. There's been a gradual destigmatisation that was long overdue.


23.

Mental illness takes up so much time. It diverts you from the life you should be living. And it's time I can never get back.

My experience has changed me. It's made me acutely aware of how mysterious and powerful the mind is. But the most important thing I've learned is this: I don't need to be afraid of my thoughts.

# Moments in This Fleeting World

## Jen McPherson

### As told to Catherine Cho

I arrive on a grey, wet February morning. The first thing I notice is the perimeter fence that encircles the low secure unit. It is about 17 feet high, dark green and made from steel. I take a deep breath and step inside. I didn't know that for the next four years, I would be living within fences like these, detained against my will.

When I first arrive at the low secure unit, I am twenty-seven years old, I am severely depressed. I am unable to think about anything but how I can end my life. Simple tasks like washing my hair or eating breakfast are a Herculean effort.

We aren't allowed anything that could be used to harm ourselves or staff; anything sharp, like tweezers or razors, is locked away in the security cupboard. However, I still find ways to circumnavigate this situation. I smuggle in a notepad and pen. I use the wire from the notepad to make deep cuts in my arms. Seeing the blood ooze out makes me feel better. It is a release.

Staff threaten to refer me to a medium secure unit if I continue to self-harm. I try to hang myself off the curtain rail, but the

37

rail collapses on top of me. I wet my fingers in the sink and jam them into a plug socket.

I stay in the low secure unit, paralysed by fear and self-loathing.

I think about everything that led me here. My psychosis started gradually. I did not wake up one day and become mad. I was twenty-three, living alone in London, and I became convinced that there were cameras in my flat. I even went out to buy a camera detector. As an aspiring journalist, I was glued to the news. The newsreaders started to make gestures towards me, and their facial expressions were directed at me. There were references in newspapers about me. I was living near to the MI6 building, and, because I had read up on counterterrorism as a politics student, I thought that the intelligence services were spying on me. I thought my every text, call and email was being monitored. I also thought that there was a global conspiracy, and I was the star of a show that everyone around the world was watching. Most disturbingly, I thought my psychiatrist had tried to drug me covertly with psychedelics, causing me to hallucinate. This went on for three years. I rarely left my flat during this time. I was in a no man's land of paranoia, purgatory and persecutory delusions. I had no insight into my illness. It was my reality.

My father decided I needed to leave London, so I moved back north. It didn't help. The delusions followed me. I thought the neighbours were plotting against me. Pretending to be on a show twenty-four hours a day for the hidden cameras was exhausting. It reached a climax when I developed a delusion that there was a tapeworm lodged in my brain and that it was slowly killing me. Someone – I suspected a local policeman – had intercepted a takeaway I had ordered and planted tapeworm eggs in my food. This delusion kept me up at night and consumed every thought during the day. I would pace around my house in the daytime and toss and turn at night. I visited numerous doctors demanding a brain scan, but none of them would give me one due to a lack of neurological symptoms. I was desperate. My brain was malfunctioning and soon I would be dead. Just like my brother. I kept remembering my brother.

When I look back to my childhood, I think of safety and love. I grew up in a leafy village, situated outside a market town. My brother and I would ride our bicycles to the cornfields at the edge of the village until dusk. My childhood was full of music lessons, sports and holidays abroad. I visited Japan and my mother's family every other summer where I would eat green-tea shaved ice with red-bean paste.

I remember my mother's Japanese curry simmering away on the stove, and my father's full English breakfast over the Sunday newspapers. Music permeated our household. I started the violin and piano when I was three years old, later taking up the viola. My brother, Ian, was a talented musician and sportsman.

Ian was my best friend, my confidant and soul mate. Four years older than me, he took on the role of protector, especially on the school bus. I was nine years old when he died. We had just returned from a family holiday in Spain, where Ian and I made friends on the beach. The next day, Ian felt sick, so my father collected him from school early. Ian continued to vomit. My father left for work, and my mother said she would keep a close eye on Ian.

What happened next would haunt me for the rest of my life. Ian appeared disorientated so I sat on his bed while my mother asked him simple questions like what school he went to. When she asked him what age he was, my brother said, 'Sixteen . . . no, fifteen . . .' He was thirteen years old. Then his eyes rolled back. Although I didn't realise this at the time, he was gone. He never regained consciousness.

My mother panicked, an ambulance arrived, and Ian was rushed to hospital. I stayed with a neighbour that evening, and it never crossed my mind that Ian would die. Death wasn't in my vocabulary. The next day, I arrived at the hospital and saw my father waiting in the corridor. I will never forget the grave look on his face. My mother appeared with a doctor, crying. 'They can't do anything,' she said, wiping away tears. She sat me on her lap and explained that Ian had died. I replied repeating the same word, 'Why?' She couldn't give me an answer. Ian had died because of a cerebral oedema. The doctors couldn't establish what had triggered it, so the cause of death was 'unknown'. My father, a Presbyterian Scotsman and a man of science, needed a cause, and he would write to doctors across the country asking them if Ian had died from various illnesses, but to no avail. My mother, a Japanese Buddhist, was more philosophical.

My father dealt with Ian's death by returning to work immediately. The grief caught up with him later in the year when he took an overdose at Christmas, which he fortunately soon recovered from. My mother put on a brave face, but I could hear her crying while running the bath every night. The death of a child is like drowning slowly; you are constantly coming up for air. There is nothing to learn from it except pain.

I flirted with madness years later in secondary school. I suffered terribly from irritable bowel syndrome (IBS) during my teenage years which negatively affected my GCSE exam results. Nothing I did would help ease my IBS. I felt like it was ruining my life. One day, I snapped. Before school, after getting off the school bus, I went to the local shops to buy two packets of paracetamol. I swallowed them one by one in the school toilets, and I remember feeling a wave of calm wash over me after I'd taken them. I went to the sixth form common room and talked to my friends as if nothing had happened. Then I started to feel nauseous; I panicked and went to the school nurse, telling her I felt sick. She made me lie down on the bed. Five minutes later I confessed to her what I had done. She called an ambulance, and the headmistress came down to comfort me.

At the hospital, they asked me why I had taken the pills and I said because I had IBS. My parents arrived. My mother cried while my father looked on stony-faced. I felt awful; not just physically, but in mental agony, too. I felt guilty for what I was putting my parents through. Shortly before discharge, the psychiatrist came to see me. My mother urged me to stress to the psychiatrist that I'd taken the tablets strictly because of my IBS. I could see that she was afraid. I returned to school the next week as if nothing had happened, and we never talked about it again. When I think about it now, I realise that was because in Japan, my mother's home, mental illness is such a taboo.

When I think of my mother, I think of her Japanese maxim, *ganbatte*, which means 'do your best'. I think of how she would feel about seeing me in this place. As much as I miss her, a tiny part of me is glad that she isn't here to see me at my worst.

It started with an itch. An itch so deep that my mother's skin would bleed from her scratching. Then she turned yellow, a symptom of jaundice. I knew deep down it was cancer. I just knew it. A few weeks later, a doctor diagnosed her with pancreatic cancer. All cancer is bad, but pancreatic cancer is particularly brutal. She recovered just in time for my A level exams, then she had gruelling rounds of chemotherapy. Remarkably, she got the all-clear while I was trekking across Nepal in my gap year.

I started university and in the summer holiday at the end of my first year, I went volunteering in Sri Lanka. My mother's cancer recurred while I was in Sri Lanka, but she didn't tell me until I had returned home. My father and I knew it was terminal this time, but we never once talked about death. I wish we had. My mother's Japanese stoicism meant she dealt with the illness by pretending she wasn't ill. Despite the toll the chemotherapy had on her frail body, she carried on driving to get the groceries right up until the very end. She never once complained or felt sorry for herself.

In the summer before she died, I had gained a prestigious internship at the *Guardian* in London. She urged me to go, saying that this more than anything would make her happy. I still feel guilty for leaving her that summer. When I returned in September, I winced at how thin she had become. She was admitted to hospital. One day she turned to my father and me, took each of our hands in her hands, and said, 'I can't do it any more. I'm so sorry but it's time.' I turned away as I choked on my tears. I asked her, 'Who will I talk to?' and she pointed to her heart.

On the day she died, my father sat in his chair next to my mother's hospital bed and read his newspaper. I held her hand and thanked her for all she'd done for me as a mother and told her repeatedly how much I loved her. A part of me died when my mother died. It was as though someone had turned off the light.

I meet with a psychiatrist. She diagnoses me with bipolar disorder. She prescribes me quetiapine, which is a mood stabiliser and antipsychotic. I stop self-harming, but it makes me feel sedated, and I gain a lot of weight in a short period of time.

I get on with the staff more than I do with the patients. Some of the patients on the ward do not like me. One in particular,

Paula, mocks my 'posh' accent. Another, Claire, tries to attack me after an argument about lending money, the latter being something that is strictly prohibited on the ward. She has to be restrained by staff. I do make one friend, Leila, a talented poet. We share books, and I give her a copy of Kahlil Gibran's *The Prophet* for her thirtieth birthday. We celebrate with a party and she has a birthday cake, without candles, because these are banned on the ward.

For the first three months of being an inpatient, I do not have any leave. I watch the other patients go outside – to meet their family, to go swimming – and I am desperate to leave. After three months, I am allowed out into the hospital grounds, escorted by staff. Stepping outside, feeling the sun on my face and breathing in the fresh, spring air fills me with unbridled joy. Eventually, I am trusted enough to be given unescorted leave. The first time I leave the ward on my own to go into town, I go to Starbucks and order a matcha latte with coconut milk. I drink it while eating a cinnamon swirl. I think, this is what freedom tastes like.

I stay on the low secure unit for just over a year and then I'm moved to a rehabilitative unit. I am still not considered well enough to leave hospital. While in the rehab unit, I start therapy with a psychologist, who asks me to call him Luke. Because of my history of self-harm, he asks that I agree to a non-self-harm contract.

Luke suggests we try a technique called imagery rescripting. We choose a negative memory that I will relive, and Luke will speak to me as if it were happening in the present. I say, 'I am sixteen years old. I take an overdose of thirty-two paracetamol tablets in my school toilets and am rushed to hospital. At the hospital, my parents arrive. I feel awful.' Luke says, 'You're just a child. How can you blame yourself when you're just a child'?

We continue, a dialogue between my past sixteen-year-old self and my psychologist. I come out of our session feeling like a weight has been lifted from my past.

Six months into my stay at the rehab unit, I relapse. I relapse because I stop taking my medication. I feel so sedated and numb, so I pretend to take it instead. I feel like it will be OK without taking my medication because the sessions with Luke are going well.

In my relapse, I rip up the flower beds in the patients' garden and throw a glass birdcage across the courtyard, smashing it into tiny shards. I write expletives across the walls with Sharpie pen. I grab a ball from the pool table and start to smash the glass window on my door. The alarms start to blare, and staff come running to my bedroom. Guy, a particularly patient nurse, talks me into sitting down on my bed and handing over the snooker ball. He steps over the broken glass, takes my hand and leads me outside to sit on the garden bench. We talk for the next hour.

He asks me about the book I'm reading, *An Unquiet Mind*. I can hear people cleaning up the broken glass in the garden.

I am wrecked with shame over my behaviour. This episode sets me back and all the progress I have made over the previous year feels lost. My psychiatrist tells me that he thinks I should go on the depot, an injection, instead of tablets because I haven't been compliant in taking my medication. I reluctantly agree. I will do anything to get better, anything to leave.

Sometimes when I am sad, I think about the trip I took to Nepal during my gap year, when my mother was well. It was the first time I had been away from home on my own. I volunteered in a remote Himalayan village, teaching English to primary school children and assisting in a playgroup with toddlers. We ate dahl with our hands and drank milk from the buffalo. My host sister would let me wear her bright magenta sari. At 5 a.m., the buffalo's tail would whack the hut where I slept, and I would wake up and walk up a nearby hill to see what a local silk farmer called the 'superview'. The sun would rise amidst the icy tips of the Himalayas, flooding the panorama with a warm orange glow. Whenever I feel sad or despondent, I think of this view and the feelings it evoked, feelings of pure wonder.

My father comes to see me once a week in the secure unit. He brings me newspaper cuttings of articles he has read that week as well as chocolates, books and banana-scented shampoo. I cry after his visits. I can tell he's wondering how we got here.

My father loved hearing about my memories of Nepal. I knew he was waiting for me to get better – after my mother died, it was just us.

My father was the greatest person I have ever known. As much as my childhood was happy, I do remember some dark times, because of my father's drinking. I think he had undiagnosed mental health problems. He was a successful patent attorney and to the outside world had a blessed life, but the first time I noticed something was wrong was the Christmas before Ian died. Ian was messing around with a chest of drawers and my father lost his temper and stormed to his bedroom. We didn't see him until after Christmas. I wondered why he'd missed Christmas dinner around the table with the rest of the family, but I knew it was because of the drink. I think my father drank to self-medicate his depression. He had a lot of trauma and loss as a child, and the drink was his way of coping with it. Looking back, I feel tremendously guilty that I didn't realise my father was suffering at the time. I was angry when he drank, but I wish I had encouraged him to seek help.

Nonetheless, we had an extremely close relationship, particularly in the years after my mother died, when he managed to stop drinking altogether. He had a terrific sense of humour and read one book a day. My father was my hero.

It is January, just before the global Covid-19 pandemic hits. I have been detained for two years now. I feel empty, devoid of any feeling or hope. It is as though a black veil has engulfed my existence. All I can think about is death and dying. I tell my psychiatrist that I want to jump in front of traffic, so he takes my leave away for my safety. A few months later, there will be no leave because of lockdown.

We enter lockdown. In the first weeks of April, my father dies from Covid. I receive a phone call from the doctor at the hospital who says that he is looking at 'end of life care' for my father. I rush to hospital to be with him. Luckily, I can stay for an hour with him as he slips away. I have to wear full personal protective equipment, which means I can't touch his skin or kiss his forehead. I feel utterly alone as my last surviving relative takes his final breaths. I wish I had made it out to see him earlier. I wish I could have one more conversation with him. I wish so many things, but it is too late.

Five days after my father dies, I wake up on my thirtieth birthday. I just want the pain to end, so I tie the belt from my robe around my neck, hoping I will pass out and die. I am put on Level 3 observations, where I must always be in sight of a staff member, even when on the lavatory or having a shower.

On the day of my father's funeral, three members of staff accompany me and I am grateful for their support. I remember my grandmother's funeral. After my grandmother died, in Japan, we went to the crematorium chamber, and when my grandmother came out of the crematorium, I was expecting ashes,

like when my brother had died. Instead, there were bone fragments, and we were given what can only be described as gigantic
chopsticks to pick the bones out of the ash and place them in
a burial urn. We then set sail from Tokyo with the urn to my
grandmother's birthplace, a remote island called Sado Island. It
felt like stepping back in time, with fishermen in their traditional
washtub boats, and fluorescent green rice paddies in every
direction. We had a traditional Buddhist memorial ceremony
for my grandmother. We laid white chrysanthemums and pushed
them out to the sea, until the brightly coloured petals floated
along to the sunlit horizon.

My father's funeral is more subdued. The seats are mostly
empty due to pandemic restrictions and there are only a handful
of us. His best friend pays tribute to him. I choose my father's
favourite music to play at the ceremony, 'Onward Christian
Soldiers', 'We'll Meet Again' and 'Auld Lang Syne'. I select
white lilies to go over his coffin. I feel so numb I can't even cry
over his death.

I remember that we all live with ghosts.

I don't miss my father too much because he loved me infinitely
when he was alive, so I have enough of his love to last me for
the rest of my lifetime.


I enter my fenced existence once again, under the watchful eye
of staff, still on Level 3 observations.

I decide that the only thing I can do while on Level 3 observations to distract myself is to watch all six seasons of *Queer
Eye*. Now and then I converse with whichever member of staff
is sat observing me; we talk about what we're watching on
Netflix, what we've eaten that day. We talk about what I need
to do to get off Level 3 observations.

Two weeks later, I come off Level 3 observations and I am

put on five-minute observations, when staff check on me every five minutes. I write in my diary, 'When I am alone, I have dark thoughts.' I tie a scarf around the door, a patient sees me and screams, 'SHE'S HANGING!' And so I am put back on Level 3 observations.

I am struggling to get out of bed. I am struggling to brush my teeth. I am struggling.

I speak to my psychiatrist, and he says he will increase the dosage of my antidepressant, Sertraline. I am now on ten-minute observations. It feels freeing to have those ten minutes to myself. Soon, however, when I am alone with my thoughts the darkness creeps in again and I start to think about self-harming. It doesn't take long until I am engulfed by a tsunami of pain once again.

I feel suicidal. I swallow batteries, and I'm put back on Level 3 observations. The staff decide to strip my room to stop me from self-harming. I am now lying in a completely empty room without any belongings, not even my clothes or books. I am not even allowed a hair clip to tie my hair back just in case I swallow it.

My psychiatrist tells me I will start lithium, a mood stabiliser. The lithium gradually works and I feel myself slowly come back to life. I look forward to starting my university course soon. The suicidal urges become fewer and fewer. I gradually come off Level 3 observations and get my belongings back. I no longer feel suicidal. I return to the land of the living. Death no longer preoccupies my every thought. I am in the light again.

When I told my father I had been diagnosed with bipolar disorder, he said: 'Well, at least it's not schizophrenia.' It says a lot about people's perceptions of bipolar disorder that it is somehow more acceptable than other illnesses. Bipolar unhinged me. Like a boat adrift from its secure mooring, it is often hard to come back to shore.

It is hard to say which is worse, the manic or the depressive phase. During mania, the filter that normally works and stops me from falling out with everyone I encounter disappears. I talk at lightning speed. I insult people. I burn bridges that are often impossible to repair. When manic, I think I am the queen of the world, and everyone else is being ridiculous. Famous people are following me on Twitter. I can solve intractable problems. Esoteric interests explode into unattainable careers. Mania is not positive; it is a place of negativity, of an unleashed beast. Depression is hellish too, but for different reasons. It is like my body is made from lead, and I literally can't move it. During a depressive phase, I remember I once looked out of the window of my flat. There was a cherry tree outside and I remember its bright pink blossom offending my sepia-tinted existence. I went back to bed. The next time I looked out of the same window, the tree was naked. Frozen. Had I really slept that long?

Life within the extremes is where I want to be. Boring is my utopia. I will never sleep through summer again.

The day has finally arrived. The day I get discharged from the psychiatric ward. It has been nearly four years since I was a free woman. I am now thirty-one years old. My body is filled with electricity at the prospect of freedom. I say goodbye to my friends on the ward, promising to keep in touch. I wonder if we will ever meet again or whether my memories of them will be confined to the psychiatric ward.

I look behind me and see the fence which has kept me enclosed for so long.

On my first night out of hospital, I sleep, and I realise it's quiet. There are no alarms. Alarms mean pain; now I am free from the pain of others. I am a person, not just a patient.

These days, I like to sit in my favourite coffee shop and watch the world go by, a world I am now part of. I no longer have to watch from the shadows. I am free.

The only thing left is guilt. But then I think, what if?

What if I forgive myself for living instead of my brother? What if I forgive myself for not being there in my mother's final weeks? What if I forgive myself for not being able to look after my father who was waiting for me all these years to get better? What if I forgive myself for my behaviour during my manias and depressions? What if all these experiences were meant to happen – the heartache, the regret, the loss? What if this is my destiny? A life with ghosts, in search of the sun.

# Skins

## Lewis

### As told to Rhik Samadder

When you hear the word 'gambling', you probably think of casinos, roulette tables, maybe horses, football, high-street bookies. I'll bet I could calculate which films spring to mind, depending on the decade you were born. *The Hustler? Ocean's Eleven? Uncut Gems?* I always knew I was too smart to get caught up in that world. I'm not one of those suckers. So how did I end up in the mess I got into? I think it had something to do with hope. There's no living without hope; it's our hardwiring. I know you're holding on to some. I hope you are.

Addicts have a grandiose relationship with hope. We mainline the hard stuff. It's not rational, but it's not without sense. Spin the Wheel of Fortune enough times, it does eventually land on $5,000. If you can stay in, there will be a transcendent moment that makes an agonising game worthwhile; that turns a nothing hand to purest gold. The infinite beauty a moment can hold: that's what we're addicted to.

Ah, do I mean that? Makes it sound pretty. When you've lost your money, destroyed your property, burnt bridges with your loved ones, there's not much pretty left. But no one starts there.

It begins in excitement. It starts with hope. Let's set the stall out straight. I became addicted to gambling when I was thirteen years old. I estimate I have gambled £30,000 of my own money (wages, pocket money, etc.) between the ages of 13 to 18.

I want you to understand this from the inside, so I'll tell you what happened to me, how this can happen to anyone. If you remember anything, remember this: video games and gambling are intertwined now. Few adults know this, and the really scary thing is that my story is far from unusual. So you need to know: this is the present and future; it's what your children are exposed to from a young age. Yet while games and gambling walk hand in hand, they are different; I think that's important to understand too.

I love games, because I love a good story. The virtual world has so much imagination. No borders, no entry criteria, total freedom of movement. What do you like? Puzzles, thrills, horror? Rhythm, religion, sports? *Town planning?* There's something for everyone. In one day I can be a soldier, a mob boss, a rebel in a magical land. I love sandbox games – walking around a totally invented world, making discoveries and meeting people, teaming up on quests. It's active, you and your choices at the centre of everything, different every time. I mean, movies are great, but why be taken for a ride if you can drive?

I think there's still an image of gamers as socially withdrawn, or something. It's decades out of date. Now we're plugged together in real time all over the planet, mic-ed up and speaking constantly. There is messaging too. People think young people all prefer messaging, but I don't. I have dyslexia, and struggle with comprehension. I use facial expression or tone to judge what people mean. Still, it's easier to message in games. You know what the other person is talking about, because it's through the playing. You're kind of in the same space. Some of you might still dismiss games, saying they lead to screen addiction, but let's be honest – how many people do you know these days who don't suffer from that?

Games got me through difficult times. Like when I had to travel to England, halfway across the world. See, I'm English but I was actually born in Australia, near Perth and Fremantle. This was the early 2000s, and my parents had relocated to be near my grandfather. Life was good there. We had a huge garden, at least it felt that way to my child eyes. Like everyone else, we had a pool. My dad was working at a plant nursery, so he created this incredible sanctuary of lavender, eucalyptus, bees everywhere. (And paper wasps, the bane of my life.) There was an area I could plant things myself, which was cool. I was outside all the time, wandering wherever I wanted. There was so much space.

My grandfather died, though, not long after I was born. When I was nine, the family decided to come back to England – a country I had never known. I lost all my friends in one move. The weather here is – well, you know. Here there's no football-field-sized gardens; you get a small patch of grass if you're lucky. My younger brother and I were sent to different schools, and had to start again. I suppose my thick Australian accent made me a curiosity, but by Year 4, everyone already had their friendship groups. They were full up. It was a puzzle I had no idea how to solve.

You lose your bearings. To make things worse, my parents separated. When you're spending alternate weekends and a day or two a week at different homes, it feels like you're always packing up, always leaving. It's tiring. It's hard, going home knowing one of your parents won't be there. Suddenly there was space around me, but it wasn't air and sky, it was a sort of distance from people and things, maybe? It was the first time I felt like there was . . . less of me, or something. I became good at being a background character.

I'm always telling myself stories, and they're not nice stories. Even now, I create rumours in my head. That if people notice me or I get something wrong, they are laughing at me, or they don't like me. I remember how when a teacher would ask me a question, I would immediately say I didn't know, even if I did. Just to shut the conversation down. If someone messages me, even just a basic message, I'm left wondering what they meant, what the emotional weight of it is. Are they being sarcastic? I look at past messages for clues. If they don't reply, I'm frantic with possibilities. Did I do something wrong? I spin out, and I hate it.

My saving grace was my younger brother. He transferred to my school, and it was good to have him there. Even just sharing a space with him made things feel more real. He looked up to me. Hero-worshipped me, almost. I could tell him how to do things, things he could listen to or watch, things he could try, and he'd actually do them. It was nice seeing myself through his eyes: someone reliable, good, worth being near.

Then I made another friend, let's call him Finn. He asked me round to play games at his house. I'd liked games before – *Crash Bandicoot*, *FIFA*, *MarioKart*, *Mario Party*, *Mario Brothers*. But we were a little older now, and graduated to light shooting games. *Call of Duty* on XBox 360 – classic mid-2000s boy stuff! It became a ritual, hanging out every Monday. It was important to me, and soon I was doing it as much as I could, sort of bingeing on it. At my dad's, there was no console so I couldn't do anything; young people mostly don't get to choose how or where they spend their time.

The gambling entered gently. It was new to me; it was new to most kids, really. It all started with a game called *Counter Strike: Global Offensive*. Basically, one team hides a bomb and the other finds it. It's on Steam, a popular PC gaming platform for developers and players. Ah, think of it as Netflix, but for gaming. Well, you can think of it like that, but it will make you seem 1,000 years old. (I'm joking! Come back!) You can buy or sell games on Steam, talk to other gamers . . . and buy useful items to help in your games. This is where the sinkhole opened up for me.

For *Counter Strike*, and games like it, you're buying skins. Skins are, simply put, graphic items that you can buy or win to alter how a game looks. They generally change the way your character or gun appear on screen. They don't make a difference to how you play, but they're cool, and half the fun. The better the weapon or cooler the skin, the more they cost. Players set the price, not designers. A cheap pistol skin might be £2. A rare butterfly knife might cost £5,000. That's not unusual. There is no upper limit – one skin sold for over £100,000. How do you think kids are competing in this kind of marketplace?

By the way, I'm telling you about this in detail because it's important. Gamers often assume adults don't understand their world. When you're a child or a teen, it feels like parents can never understand, only judge. If they knew how much money is being pumped into these games, they'd lose their minds. They might say the skins are only cosmetic, so what's the point? Yet it was only by giving the adults around me some credit, inviting them into my world, that I felt less alone in theirs.

There are three ways to obtain skins. You can play the game and you may get a random skin drop at the end of the match. You can pay the outright price that someone is selling the skin for in real money. Or, you can pay to open a virtual loot box, for a fraction of the cost of an expensive skin, in the hope of winning something good. Loot boxes are locked ammunitions crates, containing arms – but you don't know what's inside. It might be a cartel-engraved pistol, or a ruby bayonet. You have to pay to unlock the box to find out.

The slope got slippery when they introduced those. Kids mostly purchase them with credit vouchers, bought from game shops. You don't get ID'd that way, and there's no paper trail to tip parents off. Whether or not loot boxes officially count as gambling depends on where you're reading this. Each country has different criteria, different rules. But neither you nor I need a dictionary to know the definition of gambling. You pays your money, you takes your chance.

I avoided loot boxes, funnily enough, same way I never went into a bookie's. I bought my items direct, for however much they cost. Why take the risk? I was too smart for that. I still wanted those items, though. I needed them to stay competitive, and make the game more fun. And if I'm honest, they were an ego boost. These were highly prestigious items in my world, and wielding them would make anyone feel cool. You hold yourself differently, you're stronger and make better choices. Maybe confidence is another kind of body armour.

Outright gambling, of the kind you would recognise, came later. It came in waves. The first was match betting on e-sports teams. This is just like betting on real-life matches, except they're all played on computer games. I started in on that as a young teen, and I was very far from alone. This kind of betting has exploded in the last five years. During majors, matches will have many, many millions of viewers on Twitch. The offered bets were simple to start with – which team will win? Now, it's really niche. You can bet on teams to reach the semis, half-time scores, who'll score first – all the accumulators, each-ways and in-play options of any high-street bookie's. It's crazy detailed. There are a thousand ways to choose a winner, a thousand ways to lose your money.

The next wave was coin flips and jackpots. I got in deep on those. Once you try gambling out of curiosity – and all gamers try it at least once– it slowly reels you in. You start with amounts you can easily cope with losing. You might win, and get to buy the item you like. Hope wins! You might lose. You can then pay some more, or gamble again to get it back. It's so up and down, it's disorienting, but you get used to the whiplash. Keep spinning that wheel of fortune. The amounts creep up, the more you lose.

Quick games of roulette started mushrooming, everywhere. I was spending more time gambling than playing the games. I was way over my head by then. It's compulsive. It's designed to be.

The fourth wave was third-party crate sites, more expensive than those associated with the original games. These are high risk, high reward. They also let you buy skins outside of Steam, with bitcoin, PayPal, whatever. You can trade your skins according to their monetary value, buy different skins, or use them on totally separate websites. You can even cash out your skins for real money, making them a true virtual currency. So at this point the skins are nothing to do with what they were created for, i.e. improving a game. Now they're a commodity to be wagered. Chips; but not as cheap as.

Things got worse for me as my adolescence wore on. I couldn't stop. But my friends were doing it too, so it was normalised. I distanced myself from family, didn't want anyone to know what I was going through. It was the same thing almost every night; the same horrible feelings. By the time I was seventeen, I was a nightmare. I was in a low place. My brother and I had stopped spending time together; we were both hormonal teenagers, hanging out with our own age groups. We needed privacy. And maybe I didn't want to think about how I might have fallen in his eyes.

It's a terrible sensation, the moment a bet doesn't go your way. It's not one bad feeling either, but an awful cocktail of them. It's dread, first. You realise what you've done, how stupid you've been. You've just lost everything. It hits you like a panic attack, or a kind of grief. Then comes boiling anger. I was regularly having meltdowns where I would scream, smash my fist through my furniture – that's how I broke my chair, busted up my desk. The mist came over me and there'd be wheels flying off, smashing against the walls. It's scary for people that live with you. I kept all this hidden from my dad, but my mum was really upset and stressed. She'd try to calm me down, but that made it worse. The rage seemed to come from nowhere. It was followed by depression, which settled like a fog.

Loot boxes are still around, but the game has moved on again. Most games now copy the Fortnite system, which has a weekly marketplace where they release desirable items. Kids will easily spend £50 a week or more on items. They might be spending £500 a month. This is the direction they're encouraged in. There's no upper ceiling; it's a huge business and evolving all the time.

While games company methods are at best cynical, there are bad influencers too. Sponsored content is one thing: paid-for videos, YouTubers extolling how fun gambling websites are in exchange for a cheque. I can understand that. At least it's upfront. The real scumbags are vloggers and Twitchers who secretly own these sites. Twitch is a live-streaming platform where well-known gamers play for communities of fans. They're celebrities, using the platform to funnel teens towards gambling sites they profit from. They're making hundreds of thousands, even millions, paid for by the ruin of young people like me. I want to be honest about my mistakes, because I didn't make them in a vacuum. There are predatory agents in this ecosystem, whose story also needs telling.

It's not about hope any more. That's where it began, some place I can no longer remember, but it becomes about loss so quickly. Loss gathering more loss, like a rolling stone. It sucks up everything. I started asking for birthday money, not presents. I got a job in retail, cheap clothes, you'd know the place. I wasn't making much, and my pay packet would be emptied immediately. You know you're destroying yourself and wasting your life, but there's no way to redeem huge losses other than a big win, so you keep going. It's digging a series of holes, trying to get enough earth to fill in the last one. You become abstract to yourself. Sometimes I would win, and withdraw. A week later, that money wouldn't be there any more.

I left my retail job because of the anxiety and depression. I'm not in education any more, either; I couldn't keep up with my studies and I left. Under the care of mental health services, I was put on medication and had counselling. I didn't want to live. I stayed hidden in my room, my confidence completely destroyed. I'm still not in work. Those dark years took a toll.

I'll tell you what the very worst feeling was. Looking down at £100 in my hand, a birthday gift from my parents. I was thinking: 'Is that all?' In skins terms, it meant nothing. Replacing the furniture I'd broken would swallow that, never mind replacing the money I'd lost. I'd been banking on more, and now they'd ruined it. It must have shown on my face. My mother was worried about how angry I was; I was angry all the time.

It's not just the money, either – it's the loss of control, what it does to your mood and self-esteem to be unable to help yourself. You feel useless, stupid, like it's your fault. I was secretive, too. I would lie to my mum, tell her I'd been scammed, that anonymous strangers on the internet had taken advantage of me. I think she knew I was lying.

I lay down on my bed and had a vision of myself at thirty: no money, desperate, living with my mum or dad, still hurting them, still lying. I had been hiding, throwing their trust away, every day, for years, and I had nothing to show for it. Maybe the vision doesn't go far enough. Maybe they would have had enough of me, and I'd be on the street. My little brother would be a man then, maybe wouldn't even talk to me. I'd ruined my life. My dad still doesn't know the full extent of what happened, or how much I lost. I was so lonely, but I'd made it that way, and if I wanted to stop – if I was going to be saved – it would have to start with me.

And so I called my mum to my room, sat her on the bed, and . . . I told her everything. I told her I had lost an enormous amount of money during those childhood years, that I would lose the money in my hand. I had gambled all the money she had ever given me, every penny I had earned. I had nothing. She was shocked by the amount, but she didn't flinch. She told me she loved me, and would help me rebuild. She told me the birthday money was mine, the start of something new.

I don't know if I used the word addict – the truth is, that took longer to come to terms with. I had to explain it all to her, in detail, like I have to you. If parents don't understand, they can't help. I got a counsellor at CAMHS, and that was helping. But once I turned eighteen, I was discharged. I felt abandoned. There was a four-month waiting list for adult services; it's maybe a year in some places. When I finally got a counsellor, the problem turned out to be more complex. Gambling addiction support services are focused on traditional outlets: casinos and betting shops. My world was different.

Everything was virtual, all done through tradeable items or cryptocurrency – that's just how it is for my generation.

The counsellors did teach me some things. For example, that when addicts gamble, the areas of their brain that light up are the same ones that light up when you take cocaine – it is all but literally a drug. There are studies that show that the chemical imbalances, the dopamine deficiencies that lead to addiction, are in part hereditary. Yet nurture has a role, and it is almost impossible to predict who will become an addict, and to what. Everyone has a weakness. Food, sex, alcohol . . . Whatever once gave you comfort, the place you turned to when in distress, will itself become the source of distress. As storytelling goes, it's neat. As life goes, it's hell.

I stopped playing games. I couldn't see any way to keep myself safe. I was watching YouTube videos instead, over and over, feeling isolated, cut off from my gamer friends and the ways I knew to have fun. I wasn't sleeping. Those nights were difficult, and long.

I tried using imagination, the way the games did. I closed my eyes. The busted desk disappeared, the walls fell, light and sound came crashing in. I was in Tokyo, walking a crowded thoroughfare. From every side, neon signs rose into the night sky like battle pennants. An electric turquoise fell over the scene and over me, as if we had been rendered by a digital artist. Sooner or later, though, I had to open my eyes. I saw a dented desk, a screen, some books.

I have never been to Japan. I bet it's unbelievable.

So what do we do about this problem? Game developers, gambling sites, they don't care about players. They remove all the speedbumps to losing your money. We have to put them back in, laboriously. There is regulation around skins gambling in Denmark, for example, but anyone can download a VPN and pretend they're in Detroit. Raising awareness always sounded to me like a thing to call for when you couldn't make any real change. In this case, I think it's the only thing that might work. Awareness can lead to self-awareness. It has to, because the only thing that can stop an addict is themselves. And it's the hardest thing in the world.

I've met 1,000 people who have gambled, and can count on one hand those who had a positive relationship with it. I've talked to young teens all over the world. They think me and my friends are outliers, that they're not like us, because they don't have thousands to lose. In the next breath, they'll tell me how they just lost £300 of skins. I want to scream at them to stop. I want them to understand that this is how it happens.

I didn't have £30,000 either. Not all at once. It was pocket money, birthday money, Christmas money. My wages every month, gone in days. When I turned eighteen, I had access to the childhood savings my parents had set up for me, and I spent that too. I even gambled friends' money – they were using my gambling skins account as they were banned. When they were offline, I accessed £1,000 of their money and spent it. I couldn't resist. I lost everything. Well, almost everything.

My mum helped me pay my friends back. I talked openly to them about my problem. Many of them had been doing the same as me – at least they knew exactly how serious things could get. I repaid the debt to my mum, slowly, as and when I could. It was important to me. And I told my little brother.

I felt ashamed, as I unburdened my fears. I didn't want him to end up like me, someone incompetent, addicted. He told me he never stopped looking up to me. Not for one second did he think any less of me because of the gambling. He didn't want me to tell myself a story that wasn't true.

It starts with me, I still remind myself. Because one can

always find a loophole to gamble, some self-justification or method you haven't mentioned to your support network. It's boring and lonely, the slow, daily work of keeping an eye on yourself, because no one else can. With a high-street betting shop, you can self-exclude: take your photo in and leave it there, and they'll ask you to leave next time they see you. When it's just you, you have to be so clear about what you want, even if it sounds silly and basic. I wanted to keep playing games if I could. But above all, I wanted to stop gambling.

I worked out a plan with my mum. The skins I had left, I put on a website that required authentication via mobile app to access. I put the app on my mum's phone. It's behind a password I don't know. Addiction doesn't magically go away, though. It's not like the movies. I've relapsed. There are times I've created a whole new account, put some money on it, and gambled. I'm trying to strangle the urge out of me. I don't put wages into my current account now, unless it's for something specific I need. The rest goes into a savings account only my mum can access.

One day my brother came into my room, and said there was something he wanted me to see. Anime stuff he'd been getting into. It was cool. It lifted my spirits, to watch them with him. We started talking again, about other stuff. Hobbies, plans, problems in our lives. We talked about taking a trip together, where we might go. He doesn't hero-worship me, I think. He looks up to me. He knows who I am, what I struggle with, and I know the same about him. I think that's better.

I was never as alone as I felt. People saw a future for me when I couldn't. But I'm going to say it again: if addicts want to do something – thinking it will fill the hole, show them where hope is – they're going to do it. You have to readjust your thinking to give yourself self-worth. Without that, you really do have nothing.

I started trying different games again, when I felt stronger. I had seen some that reminded me of those animes we watched, ones with good stories. As well as being safe, hanging on to passion is important, otherwise you're not participating in life. I do have a few thousand in skins now, built up the hard way over several years. But I mostly avoid games with items. Temptation aside, they're very competitive and I don't feel that way any more. I want to enjoy games, and playing with my teammates. I don't want some thirteen-year-old in Omsk screaming at me that I'm a n00b.

I do look back. I could have done so much with twenty grand, laid the foundation for my future. But I accept the loss. It's gone, and gambling won't bring it back.

It's not just about the final balance. If I count the amount I won and then lost in those years, I easily gambled my way through over £110,000. And I'm small fry. I have friends who will bet £1,000 on a coin flip. I've known of young people from their teens to their twenties who have gambled half a million pounds. Ninety-seven per cent of children in this country play games. Many of them will have accounts on gambling sites – you get bonuses if you do. Young people are impressionable, and games that encourage you to buy cosmetic items rely on that. Some developers are making a billion pounds a year, with a product that fundamentally hasn't changed. They aren't designing games, they're gaming people.

I don't want other children to go through what I did, but I'm not naive enough to think the problem is going anywhere, so support services need to catch up to what has been happening, this changed landscape. Someone dies every day from gambling-related suicide, usually young men. It's not talked about. It's something I'm passionate about – if I can raise the alarm, steer things in a better direction for kids who don't have the advantages I did, the experience won't have been for nothing. I'm nearly twenty-one now. It's strange; I feel like I grew up too quickly.

I have started thinking about the future again. Whatever mine holds, I'd like it to be a good story. Top of the list is a trip my brother and I talked about when things were bad. In my imagination, I can see it: riding the shinkansen to Kyoto, eating red-bean waffles from a market, checking out gothic streetwear models. Rainbow bridges and bullet trains. Two brothers on the other side of the world, keeping each other on the path. A temple garden, in our own skins, looking out on cherry blossoms and mountaintops. So pink and hazy in the dawn light, like it was all drawn just for us.

I think that's where I'll leave you. We're saving our money, planning everything we'll need. This isn't a game, you only get one life and there's no point gambling it, because there's no bigger treasure. No one can give you more than you already have.

# Here Comes the Train

## Alain Knight

### With contributions from conversations with
### Kathryn Mannix

## On the Train

*I am waiting at the train station. The train rocks up. As the carriages pass, I see him. The same guy I saw a few days ago. This time I won't let him get away. Boarding the train, I decide to sit a few carriages behind him. My brain is bubbling like a lava lamp. I decide that I have to end all of this. I change seats and make my way down to the same carriage, checking my knife in my pocket as I move.*

*He's not dressed in military clothing this time. He's dressed like a spy, hoping I won't recognise him.*

*I decide to attack. From behind, I thrust the knife into his neck. Our arms interlock and we struggle. One of his arms drops. I thrust the knife a second time into his neck. He collapses. Grabbing his rucksack, I get off the train. Somebody confronts me. I shout, 'SAS, get the fuck out of the way!'*

*The police arrive. Standing in the bushes I wash blood off my hands. 'That's him!' shouts a bystander. I realise he means me.*

Alain is in big trouble. In fact, he's been troubled for quite a while now, but this unprovoked attack on a commuter has brought it all to a head. He's about to be arrested, to be lost in a system designed to punish criminals rather than to recognise and help people suffering from a disorder of thinking that they may not even recognise in themselves. The police will take Alain to the cells. He will be charged with attempted murder, held on remand in a prison, and his mental health will decline even further before he is eventually sent to a secure psychiatric hospital.

But let's not jump too far ahead. Instead, let's rewind to see how all this began.

Alain has lived a 'normal' life: the elder of two children, a big brother, a teen with prospects and aspirations, friends, supportive parents and grandparents. He is bilingual, thanks to his French mum and grandma and family trips to visit relatives in France. After more socialising than study in sixth form (a familiar theme in many teens' lives) he was disappointed by his exam results. Undaunted, Alain revived his career prospects by taking an HND at a local college to gain a place at university where he thrived, made good friends and acquired a girlfriend along the way.

Alain never lacked ambition. At school he'd thought about applying to Oxford University. After gaining his degree in Environmental Engineering at a university in the Midlands, he found work selling kit to decontaminate oil spills, and he aspired to be the best environmental salesman in the country. Somehow, though, those hopes were frustrated: relocating to London for the sake of his girlfriend's job, he found work in a small start-up company where he was very happy, but a merger with a bigger company led to increasing pressure against what felt like unfair odds.

Life became difficult. Work was increasingly stressful. Previously good working relationships became strained. During a 'last straw' moment when Alain felt undermined by his boss during a meeting, there was a row. Alain left the meeting, left work and didn't go back. Further trouble followed when the company demanded the return of Alain's company car and laptop, which he withheld. The police became involved. His relationship with his girlfriend disintegrated. They split up, sold their flat and went their separate ways. Alain returned to his parents' home, miserable.

## A Change Begins

*I've been out of work for nearly two years now. I have smoked away most of my remaining savings. I am living at my parents' home, which they are selling from under my feet.*

*My life milestones have all been normal so far. I know the difference between good and bad, I respect my elders and I love my family. I am polite and well mannered. Despite my recent misfortunes, I have good career prospects.*

*But things have started to change. I am stressed and anxious. I had a demanding job and fell from grace. My imagination is starting to dictate what is going on in my world. My head's a mess.*

*When I go out, I feel that people are spying on me from their homes. When I get home, I write in my diary what I saw. A lady at the bus stop wearing black, or the pattern of twigs on the ground, are signs telling me what to do.*

*I have been going to local auctions and purchasing swords. I am not sure why, but I feel the need to defend myself. Surely if they're selling swords then that's legal. But I don't think it is.*

*Today, at an auction, I see a samurai sword. It is immaculate. The sheath and handle are intricate, beautifully carved wood. I must have this.*

*The world is not safe: I'm getting prepared.*

One of the difficulties with disorders of thinking is that the disorder is not obvious to the person from the beginning. They feel unsafe because their thoughts tell them that they *are* unsafe. Yet many of us experience occasions that feel dangerous or uncomfortable, from being followed on a dark street to being undermined by a colleague at work. In retrospect, it is quite possible that some of Alain's work and relationship difficulties were because his mental illness was already beginning. Talking with him now, it's clear that some of his thoughts and ideas were very unusual. The purchase of his samurai sword was one of these. Another was his belief that he had been chosen for a very special and secret responsibility in the world.

Despite these unusual ideas about some parts of his life, Alain was still functioning normally in other parts. He had always had a close and loving relationship with his grandparents, but during the eighteen months prior to this period, both his local grannie and his grandmother in France had died, leaving him very sad. He made regular visits to his local grandad, to support him and to reduce his sense of loneliness. Alain loved these visits, which often included the treat of a shared meal of fish and chips from the local chippy, conversations and reminiscences about happy times, a shared joke and a chuckle.

It was during one of these trips to visit his grandad that Alain discovered something remarkable.


## Discovering the Treasure

*I'm housebound with nowhere to go, spending my days watching James Bond movies and believing that I too am a spy, an important spy, the head of the SAS. At night, I spy on my neighbours.*

Today is a Saturday. I leave for my grandad's mid-morning. From my parents' house the walk is about an hour and a half, so good exercise for the day there and back. My grandad lives alone now that Grannie has passed away. We all loved Grannie with all of our hearts. How I miss her.

I pick up fish and chips for both of us on the way. Grandad is entitled to OAP prices at the chip shop.

'Here he is, the intrepid traveller,' says Grandad as I arrive. We laugh as he gets out the cutlery and plates, and the salt and vinegar. We love our chip shop treat.

After our fish and chips today, I decide to take a walk up to the castle. Over the years, I've enjoyed visits to this castle with my family. It was a lovely walk there with Grandad and Grannie from their house, along the seafront. Sometimes we'd pay to visit the keep, other times we'd just walk around the scattered ruins. The whole place is full of happy memories.

On a whim, I decide to pay to visit the keep. After walking to the top of the castle and back, I find myself in the souvenir shop on my way to the exit. I'm not intending to stop here; there's lots of historical souvenirs to tempt the tourists, but I'm a local – I won't part so easily with my cash.

And then . . . my eyes are drawn to a chalice. It's sitting on the shelves, right in the middle of all the other souvenirs. It's pewter. It's important. It's staring at me. The sun dances on it, illuminating the chalice as if it was trying to get my attention. I reach out and pick it up. The goblet is heavy in my hands, hallmarked, cool and grey. As I hold it, I understand: this goblet is, in fact, the Holy Grail. All rational thoughts leave my mind. This is it. This is my purpose in life – to look after and guard the Grail.

I make what looks like an innocent purchase, yet I know that this is momentous. The Grail is in my rucksack, and I'm on my way home.

Alain is beginning to develop ideas of being special, chosen, selected for an important and secret task. Many of us might watch a spy movie and imagine the thrill of being a spy, but Alain's thoughts are more than that: he believes he *is* a spy, that he is the head of the SAS, that he has been chosen as the guardian of the Holy Grail. His disordered thinking is also driving some unusual behaviours: crawling across neighbours' gardens, posting playing cards through their letterboxes – cards that he believes indicate his neighbours' roles in an imminent crisis; and then the purchase of a samurai sword and of a facsimile antique goblet that he believes to have sacred powers.

His disordered thoughts have begun to affect his behaviour. And that is how the next trouble began.


## Losing the Plot

*It wasn't long before my interest in weapons and my deteriorating behaviour came together in what people might call an unfortunate incident.*

*I wake up late in my flat. It's just another day with nothing to do. So I eat some cereal and down a couple of cups of tea. Sometimes when I go out I wear a suit, to pretend to myself that I am still at work. But not today. Today I'm going to the pub. So it's casual top, jeans and boots. I drive to the local town and park up. This is not the first time I have risked getting into trouble for drinking and driving.*

*I have a few pints. I'm annoyed that I don't meet anyone worth talking to. I feel frustration escalating inside of me, building into a rage. I have no job, no money, no prospects, no help from the employment agency that I'm using to help me. They are useless. In my fury, I drive back to my flat, run up the stairs, collect one of my swords from the fireplace and set off back into town.*

*Damn! There's a queue on the roundabout by the motorway! I'm not waiting in a queue, I've got important business to see to. I mount the central reservation, and my wing mirror smashes into the wing mirror of another car. I just carry on and push myself into the front of the queue, then zoom across the roundabout. Checking my remaining mirror, I see that I'm now being chased by the car that I smashed into. I drive like the wind and eventually lose my tail.*

*I have one thing in mind: the staff at the employment agency have been conspiring against me. I will make them pay.*

*Screeching to a halt outside the agency's shop window, I take the sword out of the car and storm into the shop. I'm waving my sword, shouting. 'I'm sick of it!' and the staff look up, confused. I recognise the manager, and in two strides I'm holding the sword against his chest. He looks shocked, yet he remains relatively calm and brave. I sweep my sword along the desk. The movement smashes a printer and sends paperwork flying. My rage is beyond anything, driving my actions, seeking redress for the way they have ignored me, belittled me, wasted my time.*

*I hear: 'Call the police!'*

*Of course, this went to court, and I was convicted of affray and common assault with damages. Being in court was like being on the set of* EastEnders *or* Rumpole of the Bailey. *It just didn't seem real. It felt that everything was made up. I was just waiting for someone to say, 'Cut! That's it for today.'*

That boy who had big dreams as a teenager is now a young man with ideas that are distorted by a mental illness. He is still a kind, loving grandson to his widowed, lonely grandad. He still wishes he could find a job, meet someone special, hold down a relationship. But he also experiences ideas that influence his behaviour, make him feel that the world is unsafe, and because he is a kind man, he also believes that he has the responsibility to make the world safer.

The attack on the employment agency led to court and a fine. As Alain and I discuss his experiences, the irony strikes me that whilst his mind was telling him untruths that frightened him, he experienced the reality of his first court appearance as though he was trapped in a TV drama. His grip on reality was back to front. He needed help, but nobody realised.

Later, he will take the terrifying step of deciding to stab a man on a train, in the belief that the man is a public danger and that, as head of the SAS, it is Alain's job to stop him. The stabbing led to his next court experiences. This time, though, he was seen as dangerous, and was locked up for a long period of remand in prison while he awaited trial for attempted murder. He was still in need of help. Still nobody noticed.

Here's a snapshot of his life in prison.

## Banged up

*I am lying on my single bed. There's a relative stranger in a similar bed next to mine. The poky room is cold and needs a lick of paint. The windows are barred. Beyond them is a limited view of the courtyard, and tall walls and fences that are topped with barbed wire.*

*My cell is my mini-home. I have been in other cells worse than this. Leftover remains of drug usage by previous occupants dangle from the wall, silver foil on a string.*

*The first thing I hear this morning is the jingle of keys, a heavy bunch of keys. The door swings open. 'Association!' shouts the prison officer. Yes, it's real, I'm in prison. I jump out of bed still in my clothes and put my prison-issue shoes on. I'm on a mission: this is the best part of each day. A pint of cold, fresh milk is waiting for me outside my prison cell. I collect it and march down to the hot-water urn, where I fill up my flask with hot water to make my beverages. This flaskful must last me half the day; the next opportunity to fill it will be at lunch.*

*Breakfast is Coco Pops with my delicious ice-cold milk, a cup of tea* and a few morning cigarettes. Back in the cell I share with Ric, we put the TV on and chat about nothing in particular, exchanging stories. Cell-mates usually tell each other what they're inside for, but you never know whether you're being told the truth or not.

Yesterday I received my canteen order: treats prisoners can request if we have the means to pay. I've got a bar of Yorkie chocolate, some tobacco and some matches. My family sends me money every month. For £10–£15 a week you can live like a king, but you try not to draw too much unwanted attention. We can double our tobacco by lending an inmate 25 grams and receiving a repayment of 50 grams a week later. This is called 'double-bubble'. How this actually works, I don't know. I'm not sure I want to. But you have to be careful not to get too involved with other, riskier inmates. Inevitably things lead back to drugs and desperation.

Everything I need to survive is supplied: the roof over my head, my cell, the daily food, linen and clothes. It doesn't cost me anything at all. Except my loss of liberty.

Today is calmer than yesterday. Yesterday I had a squabble with my cell-mate. He had been kicking the cell door all night long. Other prisoners were shouting 'Shut up!' and I hadn't been able to sleep. He claimed to be a political prisoner, which is rubbish of course, so we argued. I snapped in the end, and I threw a cup of tea in his face. He stepped back and tried to punch me. But the screws (prison officers) were there quickly and moved him into another cell. I know this is risky for me, he has other prison friends. I could be in danger.

For inmates, the phone is the primary method of communication with the world outside. Mobile phones are forbidden and the telephone queue is always long, with friction amongst lags becoming impatient about waiting to talk to their family and friends. We have to order a phone-card to be able to make calls.

Lunch is served. We're like dogs at the racetrack as the doors are all opened. We march from the wing to the canteen. Everyone queues and *it's remarkably civilised. Occasionally there are disputes and people spill other people's meals as reprisals. The plan is to get out quickly, collect my food and get back to my cell without trouble. Once you're back at your cell, you're safer.*

Today I'm offered the use of a shower. We can't shower every day, so I'm glad it's my turn today. The showers are on the middle level of the prison, and normally two or three prisoners are allowed at any one time, with a prison officer standing at the entrance. The showers are half decent and the towels are clean but a bit ragged. It's a dangerous place, though, especially if an inmate has a vendetta. It would be relatively easy to smuggle in a small razor and attack your victim, so I get back to the safety of my cell as quickly as possible.

On Sunday evenings the screws start to round up the churchgoers. I go to the service because it gets me out of my cell for an hour or so. Maybe around fifty inmates and a couple of screws turn up at any one time.

The church is a welcome sacred space. You feel your soul being restored simply by making the visit to this holy place. There's a sense of quiet and peace in here, a longed-for break from the stress everywhere else in a prison.

The chaplain seems to be a nice man who takes his responsibilities seriously. He delivers a good sermon and is respected by the inmates, even if they're using the opportunity of reduced supervision to do small drug deals. Many people here have lived difficult lives, and this is a good place to be for anyone who wants to become rehabilitated. The chaplain offers communion. The blood and body of Christ. I wonder if he would like to talk about the Holy Grail.

After the service we are trusted to walk back to our respective cells.

Church or not, Sunday is often a day for reflection, and many inmates will think about the people we miss the most, friends and family, and the chain of events that led us here.

Sunday evening meals are important because they also contain the

*cereals for tomorrow's breakfast, and a supply of teabags. Ric and I*
*bring our meals back to our cell, and because neither of us owns a radio*
*we listen to TV to kill the time. Tomorrow beckons and we know we'll*
*do it all again, Groundhog Day style, with the additional weekday*
*activities like work details, education and gym that partly fill the endless*
*stretch of time.*

In fact, being prosecuted for attempted murder was Alain's route into skilled psychiatric help. Psychiatric reports are part of the court process, although the psychiatrist works for the lawyers and not for the individual on trial. The first time Alain remembers hearing the words 'paranoid schizophrenia' were not in a doctor's office, being offered to him with kind and concerned support, but in court as the psychiatric reports about him were read out in public.

Schizophrenia. A serious mental illness, schizophrenia affects thinking, emotions and behaviour. This was exactly what had already happened to Alain: he'd had unusual thoughts and beliefs, which triggered emotions he'd found it hard to deal with, and these led to episodes of unpredictable behaviour. One in one hundred people will be affected by the illness, and for Alain it started in his young adult life, which is typical. Also typical is his experience of stress and bereavement as triggers; the deaths of his two grandmothers within a short span of time, and Alain's work-related stresses, may have played a part.

What is less usual are his attempts to harm other people. Most people with schizophrenia, if they harm anyone at all, hurt themselves. In fact, people with schizophrenia are more likely to be hurt by other people than to cause harm. Alain, though, is one of the few whose paranoid ideas, caused by the illness, led to action with the potential to hurt someone else. He was very sick, but not receiving care and support. Instead, he was being held in the stressful environment of a prison.

The revelation of Alain's diagnosis of schizophrenia during his trial changed all that. The judge, someone Alain had not warmed to, ordered that Alain should be removed from prison and sent instead to a secure psychiatric hospital, where he would still be detained but where he could receive support, help and treatment for his mental illness. It's possible that the judge saved Alain's life. When I mention this, Alain is at pains to point out the very real life-saving actions of the paramedics who saved the life of the man Alain stabbed. There is more than one life saved, and more than one life forever changed, in this story.

A secure mental health unit is, of course, still not like living with the comforts of home. There is a mixture of residents with severe mental health problems, but the environment is less harsh than in prison, the staff are trained, specialist mental health professionals, and the purpose of the community is to restore patients to health and wellbeing using a combination of medical treatment, psychotherapy, rehabilitation and compassionate care with clear boundaries. Many patients will become well enough to leave hospital and live more independently, often in supervised, specialist hostels at first, and eventually in their own homes.

Alain will not be permitted to return home until his trial is concluded, his sentence pronounced and served, his thinking and behaviour restored to a state where he is safe, and until he poses no more threat to other people than an average citizen might. He has a long road ahead.

## Living in a Psychiatric Hospital

*Breakfast has come and gone on the Continuing Care Ward. The choice always seems to be either cereal (porridge, ironically) or a bacon* sandwich. *We have an early smoke. We are always clucking for our nicotine fix.*

It's ward round day, 9 a.m., and I'm as ready as I'll ever be. The MDT (multi-disciplinary team) consists of a psychiatrist, psychologist, occupational therapist and nursing staff. To walk into a room with all these professionals who have a say in your life is truly daunting. Ward rounds only happen every two weeks, and they are patients' only opportunity to advocate for ourselves and understand what our medical team wants from and for us. I know how much is riding on this morning's meeting. I have been waiting two weeks for a decision about my application to have escorted walks in the hospital grounds. Currently, I'm limited to watching the sky through the windows because I have no approval to stand in the fresh air.

As I enter the room, there is quiet. I sit in the 'Mastermind' chair, ready to answer questions and even ask a few myself if I'm not too intimidated. The OT lady is doodling on her notepad whilst the nurse chairs the meeting. How have you been? We hear you've started playing badminton and table tennis. We would like you to start the emotional regulation group therapy once a week on a Friday. *They approve my escorted ground leave for fifteen minutes a day. I feel a rush of relief. I have been in this secure hospital for about six months. I have a long time yet to go. You hear about people who are discharged via tribunals, and this gives me hope. One day that will be me.*

It's still early morning when I leave the meeting room. I sit down in one of the ward's communal lounges. Frank is sitting opposite me. He looks a bit agitated; he's just got out of bed and has had no breakfast. His ward round is in a minute and he is waiting to be called forward.

The successful formula for preparing for your ward round is to get up earlier, wash, wear something smart, have breakfast and have a couple of cigarettes. The ward round conversation may be incredibly short — ten minutes is good going. At least if you prepare, you have a chance of things going in your favour. Frank clearly hasn't set himself up for his meeting.

Frank is called in. I sit and think about our experiences here. Sometimes the ward round feels like a bit of a game, an opportunity to tick boxes and prove you are well. But my life is at stake. I am surrounded by unstable and in some cases dangerous patients. The staff are administering medication to me, recording and watching my move-ments and activities, expecting me to engage in group and one-to-one therapy. I didn't choose this, but maybe this is a result of my actions. I'm not even sure if I'm the same person any more. I crossed a line when I committed my offence, and I don't think I'll ever be the same.

Frank comes out of the ward round room. There are raised voices, shouting. 'Bastards have removed my community leave,' he says to me and a few other patients that have since come into the lounge. 'Fuckers are taking my CDs away too!' Frank returns to his room with two staff following him. I watch him go and reflect that in this secure hospital, although it's not quite a prison, a lot of the time it does feel like it is Us and Them.

It's still Tuesday morning and it's medication time. Patients queue at the medication hatch. Staff round up any shirkers. Rob is arguing about his medication being too strong; he's saying that the medication makes him tired. The staff placate him, trying to get his co-operation and compliance.

We roll into lunchtime. This is a welcome break as we get off the ward and walk down to the canteen, where another queue forms. Unlike prison, the food here is truly terrible. But some people like it, and the canteen staff argue that most service-users smoke and can't taste food properly anyway.

After lunch, my psychologist turns up to see me. We have been meeting weekly. The other patients wolf-whistle and laugh — juvenile behaviour is common. 'Your girlfriend's here, Al!'

So here we go again with the psychologist. Raking over my offence *yet again. We start with the pleasantries:* How are you, what have you been up to since we last met? Let's talk about your family and friends today. *I say that my life is being wasted here, while my friends on the outside all have successful lives. We discuss what roles and relationships I have. It feels like I do most of the talking. In fact, I feel that I could be talking to a robot for all it seems to matter.*

*Now that I've finished my psychology until next week, I do some reading in the quiet room. I crack on with my* Dragon's Den *book, dreaming of becoming a successful businessman once I get out of here, while those patients who have small jobs, like ward representative, clothes shop assistant and librarian, leave the ward to attend to their responsibilities.*

*Sometimes things kick off. The alarms go. A fight, or some vandalism. This is normal, and security is tight. Today we are rounded up into the main lounge. The staff explain that they are going to do a ward and room search. A metal fork from the canteen has gone missing. One by one we are frog-marched to our respective rooms where we are patted down and then a couple of staff go through the room and all our belongings. This process takes an hour and a half. Sometimes they find what they're looking for, sometimes they find other contraband, and sometimes they don't find anything. We patients are annoyed by the invasion of privacy, often caused by the irresponsible behaviour of the same repeat offenders.*

*It's time for tea. Hot dogs in rolls with onions. Quite popular. But it doesn't really fill you up. By eight o'clock I will be hungry again.*

*Twice a week the gym runs in the evening. I don't go. I find it hard to smoke twenty a day and then go on the treadmill for thirty minutes. Nevertheless, the sporting facilities are quite good. Five-a-side football, badminton, table tennis and soft tennis. The gym annex has cardiovascular equipment such as treadmills, cross-trainers and exercise bikes. Unlike prison, there's no weight-lifting equipment: the staff might struggle to manage if a bulked-up patient was unwell enough to need restraint for their own safety or the safety of other patients.*

*Finally evening medication, the last cigarette of the day and some well-earned sleep. Having my own room is a huge advantage over prison. I have survived one more day.*

In our conversations preparing this chapter, Alain's path out of paranoia and delusion slowly became apparent. It's very hard for people with a mental illness to notice when their thinking changes, and so it was following the changes in Alain's behaviours, and the shift in his focus from himself to the difficult plights of other patients, that shone a light on his recovery.

When he arrived at the secure hospital, Alain was willing to accept medical treatment: the drugs he was prescribed, despite their side effects, gradually reduced his paranoia and the grip of his delusions began to loosen. In the early days in hospital, he saw compliance with treatment as a game, as ticking boxes and avoiding prison. Yet his observation of Frank, a disturbed patient still unable to prepare for his own ward round conversation, and the compassion with which Alain reflected on that episode, shows that the kind young man inside him was gradually taking over from the head of the SAS. He was reorienting to reality, and he would make a point of welcoming new patients, recognising their fears, helping them to settle into their new environment.

That wish to help has continued and grown. Since his discharge from the secure unit, via intermediate and rehabilitation care, and now living in a house of his own, Alain has continued to help other people living with life-changing psychiatric illnesses. He is employed by a mental health NHS trust, and he uses his communication skills and personal experience

81

to support, encourage and help patients who are still fragile, vulnerable or frightened.

We talked about his sorrow for the pain and trauma he caused to the man he stabbed. Alain lives with his remorse for that act. I was interested to observe that, no matter how often he helps other people to understand that their behaviours while they were deeply deluded and paranoid were a result of their illness, he still feels guilt about his own actions. He would have liked the opportunity to meet and to apologise to the man he stabbed. An opportunity was raised by the team that negotiates such meetings in the interests of 'restorative justice', but the man Alain hurt declined his offer. Alain regrets, too, that his plea of 'not guilty' of attempted murder made his victim's mother feel anxious that perhaps the wrong man had been arrested. It seems to have been her tenderness that moved him. It matches a tenderness I have observed in Alain over the time we have worked together.

There's an unrealistic public anxiety about the idea that people with a diagnosis of schizophrenia are not locked away for public safety. We're all in more danger from 'healthy' people who are drunk or driving unsafely than from an attack by an unidentified person with a mental illness. It's been a real privilege for me to get to know Alain, to hear his story and to observe how valiantly he has worked to re-establish a normal life from the wreckage brought about by his illness. He's aware that, although life hasn't gone to plan, he has the opportunity to live well in the future. He remains in touch with old friends made before his illness and during his recovery; his family are supportive and engaged; he enjoys his job.

And one day, he'd like to live in the south of France. I'll be going to visit, if I'm invited.

# You Only Live Twice

*My two alarms and phone all synchronise to wake me up. It's 6 a.m. and it's a Wednesday. I curse as I make a huge effort to roll out of bed. I am hung-over, not from beer but from my antipsychotic medication. A Mr Grumpy T-shirt wouldn't do me justice.*

*I work part-time for an NHS mental health trust, and today is a work day. Here's the morning routine: medication for my diabetes and blood pressure, a lateral flow Covid test that takes fifteen minutes. Negative. Thankfully, I enter the result on my work computer.*

*Next, a shower. No need for permission, escort, patting down. I am at liberty. I am living alone, and I have planned my day ahead.*

*The taxi ride to the station takes about fifteen minutes, then I try to snooze throughout the forty-minute train journey. I always think that one day I might see my victim on the train or waiting on the platform. I am always slightly nervous. I would apologise for the hurt and inconvenience I have caused him and his family. But that wouldn't be enough.*

*The train rolls into the station, I wait to be picked up and after about twenty minutes, John, my line manager, pulls up in his Citroën. I jump in and off we go. Our itinerary for the day varies: sometimes we visit community patients, sometimes we go to the office, sometimes we have my supervision session. This is a responsible job and all staff working in mental health have supervision to support us in helping our patients.*

*I normally eat my sandwich in the staff kitchenette with a cup of tea. Lunch is important, especially as I have diabetes and I'll need the energy to cope with a long day. I can decide when I eat. A tiny, enormous freedom.*

*In the afternoon I help with the transition group. This is a group of patients who are transitioning from secure hospital into community accommodation. The programme I help with offers modules designed to* support them to adjust to living in the community again, to cope with the anxiety of living outside the supportive boundaries of the hospital, and to decide how much of their mental illness story to share with other people, whether new friends or future employers. Our discussions include topics like Emotional Regulation, Disclosure, Budgeting, Health and Wellbeing, and Community Survival.

Today I am the peer support worker in my role. Although I'm here as an adviser and educator, I will also learn today because every day is a school day, but the focus is on our service-users and not on me any more. I make hot and cold drinks for the patients that have turned up for the group. Anita says that she doesn't want to stay for the duration of the presentation today. That's OK, we say. The fact that she has made it at all is a positive. I notice that this girl has extensive scarring on her left arm. She is extremely vulnerable; I hope we can continue to help her. The others contribute during the talk. We give today's presentation and then run some group exercises like colouring to music (teaching people skills to soothe their own anxiety), listing main expenditures to learn budgeting, and mindfulness. We wind up the session with feedback forms.

I get a lift back to the train station, and take the bus from my local station back to where I live. I consider what to have for my evening meal. Sometimes I cook, or I might get a Chinese takeaway. Then I write my notes and observations for the patients I have met today. Once, staff observed me. Now, I am observing patients. It's important that people's progress is observed and encouraged, and any difficulties are noticed and addressed as early as possible. I reflect on how my perspective has changed. I email my notes to my line manager and that's the last effort of the day. It's about 6 p.m.

Today I have helped people. I have made a small contribution to their wellbeing. I identify with what they're going through, they become my buddies and we face a recovery journey together.

When I'm not at work, I adore my free time. I try to keep well both mentally and physically. Work provides intellectual stimulation and I try to go swimming regularly to help with my diabetes. I'm still under a Ministry of Justice Mental Health Act, Section 41 Order conditional discharge (which means I am still under supervision as an outpatient for my mental health, and if my mental health deteriorates in a way that might put me or the public in danger, I can be sent back to a secure hospital with or without my agreement) and I have a tribunal on the horizon.

My mental health recovery journey has not been straightforward. We are all different in one way or another. We all need different types of help. I am lucky my antipsychotic medication seems to work for me. My symptoms don't linger so much. I have community help, a psychiatrist, a care co-ordinator and I work with mental health professionals. I hope and pray that my good health continues and that I can live a meaningful life.


## Postscript

On 1 December 2022, at a mental health tribunal, I was awarded an absolute discharge. My application was supported in person by my psychiatrist and my social worker. My freedom has been given back to me, eighteen years after I committed the offence on the train.

# They Can Just Fuck Right Off

## Jeremy Gavins

### As told to Tracy Chevalier

He was Jeremy and he was a happy boy.

He became Jerry, hiding Jeremy behind a rough wall, and he was miserable for decades.

Now he is Jeremy again. Late sixties, gruff, blunt, very Yorkshire. Big white beard, beer belly, wears black. Dog always at his side. Lives alone in a two-up two-down in Cumbria. Builds walls in the Lake District, his rattling Land Rover stuffed with tools, smelling of dog. Goes to his local pub most nights. Signs off Cheers and Beers.

Jeremy is also open and vulnerable and can't understand why people like him. He cries easily over his own story.

This story has a happy ending. Of sorts.

## Young Jeremy

1960s Yorkshire childhood in Keighley. Mother, father, third out of four brothers. Playing outside with the kids in the street. Catholic household, Mass every Sunday. His mum cooking in the kitchen, hanging out laundry in the back garden, hoovering in the lounge. His dad in the cellar, making puff-puffs, model steam trains and traction engines he takes to shows. Uses plenty of electricity to make them, but he won't let anyone else turn on appliances and run down the meter. Mean old bugger. No central heating, add another jumper.

His dad was going to go to university, he was that clever. But the Second World War started and he fought and when he came back, no more university for him. Work. Always work. Manager at the local employment exchange. He hates the unemployed. Later he hates Jeremy going on the dole. He hates a lot of things about Jeremy.

His parents never hug their sons. They switch off the telly if there's a whiff of sex on the screen. Even David Attenborough nature programmes are too much. If his father had been Noah, there would have been only one of each animal boarding the ark.

Jeremy's escape plan: he will do his A levels, go to university, find his freedom away from Keighley.

Age eleven he discovers boys' bodies. Out in the woods, playful, experimenting. He is not the only one.

What's his favourite book at the time? The illustrated Bible, with pictures of half-naked men to look at without guilt. Just reading the Bible, Dad.

At Catholic grammar school in Bradford, Jeremy becomes a foul-mouthed, rufty-tufty rugby player, becoming a bit of a Jerry, disguising his true self. No one knows he's attracted to other boys.

God is good, his mum says so often it's almost a verbal tic. As an adult he tells her, Mum, every time you say that, I'm going to say fuck off.

There is a lot of Catholic Church in Jeremy-Jerry-Jeremy's

story. The damage it does to one life. To many lives. How is it possible to forgive?

Fuck off.

## The Most Beautiful Boy

Jeremy has told this part of the story many times before, to friends, to family, to strangers, to therapists. At the pub, on the radio, on telly. He tells his story as he sits out with a writer by a dry stone wall they're repairing in the Duddon Valley, the most beautiful valley in the Lake District. Fifty years on, he still cries over what was done to him. The tears are part of the telling. But it helps to tell it; it's what humans do. When we tell stories, we reshape what has happened to us into something we can control and analyse and make safe. Defusing the bomb by taking it apart.

Stephen is the most beautiful boy in Jeremy's school. Slight, black hair, looks like the singer Donovan. In 1968 he turns up in class and fourteen-year-old Jeremy thinks: *Ooh, he's gorgeous.*

They become mates, good mates. Two years of being good mates before Jeremy gets up the courage to tell Stephen he loves him. Stephen's response? 'It's about time! I thought you were straight.' No calling him queer, no disgust, no rejection. Just affirmation.

For the next two years they are outwardly mates, secretly a couple. Jeremy is in love and a happy boy. He and Stephen in the only gay pub in Bradford, lifting pints; Jeremy can't stop looking, lovestruck. Singing Diana Ross songs together. The pinnacle of his life reached so quickly. Maybe too quickly.

You could say it's Stephen who first swings the wrecking ball at the idyllic dream house Jeremy has built of their relationship. That beautiful black-haired boy doesn't realise the havoc he's about to wreak. Spring 1972, one night at a party in Leeds, a bit of dope smoked, he casually says: 'When school finishes we'll be going our separate ways. We might not see each other again.'

Jeremy has had two years to think of this himself, but he has not thought of it. Because he's been too busy and happy living in the moment, the beautiful present, with the beautiful boy beside him. Why think ahead? But Stephen is different. He's arty-farty, doing languages, he's making plans, going places (Paris) that don't include Jeremy. Stephen plants this seed of the future in Jeremy, a future without his beautiful boy. Stephen himself does not seem bothered by this future; Jeremy has always wanted and needed him more than the other way around.

Now Jeremy is confused, upset, worrying about the future when he's never had to think too much about it before. It doesn't help that he's taking A levels shortly. The pressure is on.

One day in class it finally gets to him. Jeremy gets up, walks out, sits against a wall in the corridor, cries. A teacher who is also a priest comes by and asks him what's the matter, takes him to his study, sits him down, concerned, sympathetic, especially when Jeremy says he's worried he'll fail his A levels.

Then he confesses he's in love. Still sympathetic, the teacher says, 'We all fall in love. Why cry?'

'Because it's with Stephen', says Jeremy.

If he hadn't said Stephen's name, he might have gone on to have a very different life.

But he says it, and the teacher completely changes, sympathy gone, replaced with anger, disgust. Now he's sent to the headmaster. Now he has weeks of haranguing, of comments about how disgusting he is to lust after men, how sinful and diseased he is, how he will go to Hell. Weeks and weeks of this.

Jeremy is eighteen, an adult, so parents don't need to be involved. Stephen is seventeen, which may be why the school doesn't go after him too, because they would have to bring in his slightly more liberal parents who might not agree with them and what they want to do. For the headmaster has a plan. 'We can't have homosexuals at this school', he says to Jeremy. 'You have a choice. We will expel you, and you won't take A levels. Or we can send you to be cured, and you'll still be able to sit your exams.'

What sort of choice is that? The sort of choice where you want to say:

Fuck off.

Jeremy doesn't say fuck off. He hasn't yet got the courage to say it. This is 1972, not 2022. The world is still dominated by homophobia, and his world by the Catholic Church. Instead, he agrees to the treatment. He wants to sit his exams and get the hell out of Keighley.

The headmaster tells him to visit his GP and ask to be cured of homosexuality. This is 'consent', though he has no idea what he's consenting to, what the treatment is.

A priest accompanies him to his first session at what Jeremy dubs the loony bin, half a mile up the road from school. After that he is to take himself to the sessions. A psychiatrist interviews him, asking him detailed questions about what he's done with other men and boys. Getting plenty of detail, always lots of detail about the sex. Then he explains they're going to give Jeremy electric shocks to cure him of his feelings. Aversion therapy, he calls it. Conversion therapy, it's now known as.

The next session Jeremy goes to the loony bin and has to take off his clothes and wear a dressing gown and slippers. They strap him to a chair, attach electrodes to his right forearm, give him a button he can push with his left hand if the shocks get too painful. That left button rarely works. The doctor leans forward and opens Jeremy's dressing gown. So he can see him.

He is facing a big screen, and they start projecting images of naked people onto it. When a naked woman comes up, nothing happens. When naked men appear, Jeremy is given a painful electric shock, like touching an electric fence except worse, because it's no accident. Burning, stabbing, Jesus fucking Christ! A pain he never gets used to.

Yep, it's really that crude; treatment a five-year-old would make up. And it is administered by the NHS.

Jeremy has sessions two to three times a week for six months. Does it work?

Fuck off.

The distinction between naked women and naked men is completely lost in the treatment. When Jeremy sees a picture of a naked woman, he's not thinking, *Oh, relief, that's good*. He's tense, thinking, *Oh no, next there will be a man and I'll get a shock*. The anticipation of pain is almost as bad as the pain itself, and it extends over all the photos, over all the sessions, over the whole six months, over his whole life.

After that first session, Jeremy walks back to school and *takes an A-level exam*. That is how it's been scheduled by his school, by the teachers, by the priests who say they care. He sits in front of the exam, and cannot get his hands to stop shaking. After half an hour, he leaves.

That term he fails all his A-level exams, except the one he did before aversion therapy started.

Jeremy has been banned from seeing Stephen. They do manage to meet twice, when exams are almost done. Stephen is backing off; he doesn't want to go through what Jeremy is going through. He has always been less involved, and soon he'll be gone. The last time they meet, he gives Jeremy a pentagram he has made out of lead. For protection.

School has Jeremy return in the autumn to repeat the year and resit his A levels, which he fails again – except for Chemistry, passing with a D. No university. That will not be his escape from his upbringing.

For a few months of that repeat year, he continues with aversion therapy, the school holding out the threat of telling his parents and expelling him. The sessions shift a little. Maybe they're getting desperate because the photos of naked men haven't worked. Now instead of showing him pictures, they ask him specifically about Stephen. Do you think about Stephen? Yes. *Zap*. Imagine yourself in bed with Stephen, are you picturing it? Yes. *Zap*. Do you love Stephen? Yes. *Zap*. They ask for a lot of detail.

Jeremy finds ways to insulate himself from the pain. He detaches himself from his physical body, floats away. He goes inside his head and makes up stories to lose himself in, stories about him and Stephen. The treatment actually has the opposite effect of what was intended: it makes his and Stephen's relationship even more important than it might have been. Stephen becomes the love of Jeremy's life. Still is, fifty years later. An obsession of sorts.

Here is one of the stories. Stephen rings Jeremy and asks to see him. Jeremy is overjoyed, and catches a train to the bus stop where they are to meet. He can still picture the snow that day, Stephen getting off the bus and running across the road towards Jeremy. He slips, and is hit by a car, dying right in front of Jeremy. The love of his life is dead. It is so vivid that Jeremy believes it. For forty years he believes Stephen died in the snow in front of him.

Six months in, the treatments stop. Something happens, something that Jeremy is still fuzzy about. Many years later when his mother dies, he reads her diary for 1972 and discovers he was hospitalised for three days. Possibly they took the treatment too far, gave him shocks that were too strong, and he passed out. Whatever happened, it scares them off.

Where have his parents been during all this? In the cellar, in the kitchen. When Jeremy – maybe Jerry by this time – uses the word 'gay', they say, 'You've ruined a perfectly good word.' They say, 'Don't bring that filth into this house.'

When Jeremy reads his mother's diary for 1972 he also finds out she knew about the aversion therapy when it was happening, and his father must have too. Jeremy has always assumed they didn't know; the school told him they didn't, and they never said anything about it. If they knew, they might have stopped it. What parent would agree to putting their child through such an ordeal?

Religious parents who switch off the telly when sex is hinted at. Who never hug their children. Who think homosexuality is a sin. Who think it's more important to 'cure' their son of homosexuality than to help him pass his A levels and go to university. That's who.

Parents a failure. The Catholic Church a failure. NHS a failure.

You can just fuck off.

Forty-five years later Jeremy does not attend his father's funeral.

To be clear: the aversion therapy does not work. Jerry is still attracted to men rather than women. Not long after he finishes school he publicly comes out, and for a while he sleeps with a lot of men (he tries with women but it doesn't work, though he prefers them to men as friends), and has a couple of short relationships. What the treatment does do, though, is to make him averse to love. He clings to his love for Stephen like a lifebuoy, as he does to the pentagram Stephen gave him. But aversion therapy keeps him from finding other loves. Eventually he goes off sex and becomes celibate.

Other smaller side effects from the treatment: he can't wear slippers or dressing gowns or watches or buttoned cuffs. He has shooting pains or itching in his right arm. He never goes to the cinema.

That is the 'success' of aversion therapy: aversion to slippers, gowns, watches, cuffs, cinema. And love. What a success.


## Becoming Jerry

That is the core of Jeremy's story, one he's told many times to many people. The story that changes his life, and turns him from Jeremy into Jerry.

Every story has a beginning, a middle and an end. The middle part is the Jerry part, and it's full of anxiety, depression, drink, panic attacks, accidents, suicide attempts. Job-hopping, restlessness, physical and mental chaos. All the stuff that emerges from those traumatic six months of pain. The stuff that makes him start calling himself Jerry rather than Jeremy.

Once Jeremy is openly gay – at least in the Bradford gay scene – he has fun for a while, but eventually finds little satisfaction there. At that time the world is too homophobic for him to feel safe and comfortable. And his family, the Church, the aversion therapy have all done a number on him, convincing him that Jeremy is bad. After a while 'Jerry' emerges, rougher and tougher, and begins to hate the Jeremy part of him for being weak and untrustworthy. In Jerry's eyes, Jeremy betrayed Stephen by admitting his love to others. *Call me Jerry*, he thinks now. *I am not Jeremy. Only people who hate me call me Jeremy*. Teachers, parents, priests, doctors. Jerry hates them all.

He no longer looks for sex or any kind of close connection; he becomes hardened. He jumps from job to job: textile factory, railway, teacher (briefly), volunteer conservation work. It isn't all bad. He has lots of good times, he thinks. He begins rock climbing. He walks in the Lake District. And he drinks, so much he damages his liver. Jerry feels at his best when he's working alone, or walking alone, but he does work with others, climbs with others, drinks with others. And the thing is, people like him, they think he's good company. He *is* good company. Jerry doesn't understand why, for he's not being honest, he's hiding his true self. 'Jerry' sits in the pub for hours, joking and laughing with others, but walking home alone, 'Jeremy' is in pain.

All this time – years and years – he thinks about Stephen, whom he still loves and whose death he thinks he's caused. Every now and then Jerry breaks through the wall he's built to hide behind and tells someone – usually a woman – about his past, about Jeremy and Stephen. Eventually it catches up with him, all this hiding and shoving down feelings. He has to deal with what happened to Jeremy, twenty-five years late.

Three things help him to do this, and Jerry to become Jeremy again: dogs, dry stone walls and therapy.


## Dogs

Jeremy's dog Timmy goes everywhere with him. To work, to the pub, on the sofa watching telly, asleep in the same bed. A border collie mixed with mongrel, he has bright brown eyes and no mean streak. He will chase a ball for hours and rarely tires. He is a happy, eager, loving presence. Jeremy has had him for ten years, and before him, another dog, Boady, for twelve years.

The thing about dogs is that they love you unconditionally. They always want to be with you. Timmy sits as close as possible to Jeremy at the pub. Sometimes he sits on him. It's an effective, therapeutic ego boost.

Dogs don't judge – or if they do, they forget it a minute later. Their attention spans are short.

Dogs live in the moment. They don't dwell on the past, as Jeremy has for fifty years. They don't worry about the future. They just want you to throw the ball, feed them, take them for walks. Timmy has brought Jeremy back into living in the present the way he did when he was young.

Dogs never say, 'When school finishes we'll be going our separate ways. We might not see each other again.'

They never say, 'You are sinful and disgusting and you will go to Hell.'

They never say, 'Don't bring that filth into this house.'

They never zap you.

They never betray you.

Once Jeremy gets a dog, he stops travelling abroad or very far in the UK. He's a homebody now in his two-up two-down that he's recently painted red and green. Timmy's constant presence steadies him. And Timmy depends totally on him, which means Jeremy can't abandon him; if he kills himself, the dog won't understand where he's gone.


## Dry Stone Walls

Jerry works at a lot of different jobs. He has been so unhappy that nothing really sticks. But somewhere along the way he learns how to build walls. Literal walls, though he has built his share of figurative walls too.

Dry stone walls are made of stones from the land, laid on top of each other, overlapping, without mortar holding them together. The stones aren't reshaped in any way with a hammer or chisel. You use what's there. Larger stones for the bottom layers, smaller as you build up, stones laid on the top in vertical or slanted or horizontal patterns that encourage the rain to run off.

You see dry stone walls mainly in the north – Yorkshire, Lancashire, Cumbria, Northumberland. Stark grey lines running up and down the hills, dividing land into fields, keeping sheep and cows in or out. They are beautiful, rugged works of art. Very practical. An essential part of the northern landscape. They're timeless, they're what our ancestors would have seen. A well-built dry stone wall lasts for hundreds of years, with the odd repair here and there.

At first when you look at dry stone walls you think the stones fit together perfectly. Look more closely and you start to see gaps. If you ever make one, you quickly realise the stones don't fit perfectly at all. Often you have to wedge them with smaller stones to stabilise them. Jeremy says there's no such thing as the perfect stone, there's just the stone that fits well enough. And you don't think about anything else while you're building it other than, *Which stone next? Will that fit?* It is deeply satisfying work.

Jeremy goes out in his Land Rover with Timmy to work on walls in beautiful parts of the Lake District. There are few people around. Sometimes he works with a partner – a woman he has known for years and trusts. Often he's on his own. It's perfect for him – no boss telling him what to do, minimal interactions with others, just him and his dog and the land and the stones.

When he was younger he could build 8 metres a day. These days he's slower and works shorter hours and builds 2 metres a day. He could retire but he likes it too much. In forty years he has built 16.5 kilometres of wall.

It's tempting to use dry stone walls as a metaphor for Jeremy's story. He is the stone that doesn't fit into the space his parents and the Catholic Church make for him. Aversion therapy is the attempt to shape him into the stone that will fit. None of us fits perfectly but if we stack ourselves right, with wedges to help, we make a solid wall. Et cetera.

But that is taking a decent metaphor and trying to fit it into the perfect space. We're not going to do that. We're not going to do what the Catholic Church tried to do.

Fuck off.

## Therapy

Dogs and walls help you live in the moment. But Jeremy's trauma lies in the past, and until he deals with that, he will never really move on, but will suffer from flashbacks, panic attacks, breakdowns, depression.

There are a lot of therapies out there for trauma. Jerry tries many things over the years, talks to GPs and counsellors and therapists, takes pills, self-medicates with alcohol. Twenty-five years after the aversion therapy, he has a mental breakdown and receives forty psychotherapy sessions over two years, half of which are for bereavement counselling over Stephen's death.

Finally, an astute therapist says, 'You have PTSD'. Post-traumatic stress disorder. Here is a diagnosis that makes sense. PTSD is often used to describe the responses soldiers have to war situations. Jeremy went through a six-month war with the

Catholic Church, his school, his parents, the NHS, and it has left him with PTSD for decades.

Eventually Jerry makes an incredible discovery about what his brain has done to protect him. One day during a session, he has a sudden feeling about the memory of Stephen dying in the snow in front of him: maybe the memory isn't real. Maybe his brain made up the story of Stephen's death to disconnect Jeremy from reality, killing his attachment to Stephen by killing him off in his head, protecting him by giving the aversion therapists what they wanted.

Eventually Jerry goes online and tracks Stephen down. However, this is no romantic story where the lovers lose touch and then rediscover each other years later on social media. This is not the happy ending everyone may be craving. It turns out Stephen *is* dead, but he died in 1983, eleven years after Jerry thinks he did. Soon after A levels Stephen moved to Paris, came back, lived in London, then Blackburn, and eventually died in a car crash.

All that bereavement counselling was for an imaginary death.

How to respond to the realisation that your brain has lied to you all these years as a way of protecting you?

Another therapist suggests he try EMDR: Eye Movement Desensitisation and Reprocessing, a therapy sometimes used for people suffering PTSD. EMDR is based on the theory that trauma can sometimes cause memories not to be processed by the brain. They get stuck and result in the person suffering from depression, anxiety, panic attacks, suicidal thoughts, self-harm, addiction. To unstick them, you picture the traumatic memory while looking from side to side or having your head or body tapped on each side. This seems to connect two sides of the brain, which makes it possible to process those negative feelings. It sounds a bit daft, and no one really knows why it works for some people. But it works for Jerry. It allows him to process the story of Stephen's death, to see it for what it is – a fantasy to protect Jeremy. It makes it easier for Jerry to come to terms with what has happened to him, to give him some closure.

The therapist also helps him to prize his love for Stephen, and it was Jeremy who Stephen loved, not Jerry. That understanding makes it easier for Jerry to go back to being Jeremy again.

## Jeremy Again

You don't go from being sick to being well overnight. It's not black and white, there are plenty of grey days, days when you're still furious at the Catholic Church, at your parents, at the NHS doctors who did this to you. Days when you cry. Nights when you go to the pub for the pints, not the company. Plenty of Jerry days.

The doctors, the Church, the school told him for months that he was a diseased, sinful boy. However much he resisted it, some of that message has sunk in. Jeremy has found it hard to understand what his friends see in him. He hasn't trusted many people. He is still wary. He has never fallen in love again, doesn't want a loving relationship.

But he's more honest now. A few years after the EMDR therapy, he writes a book about his experience of aversion therapy. Telling his life story so that he can take back control of it. He tells the farmers he works for, the people he knows in his local pub. His brothers. He goes on the radio, he goes on the telly. He becomes something of a spokesperson for banning conversion therapy.

People are horrified by what he has gone through. They also accept him as he is. The world – parts of it at least – is a very different place from 1972. Gay has gone mainstream, is unremarked upon. At times it's even a badge of pride. Jeremy's enlightened nieces love telling people their gay uncle builds dry stone walls. He wears a T-shirt to one of their weddings that reads 'I am the rainbow sheep of the family'.

Conversion therapy, however, is still with us, though there's little evidence that it works. Shock treatment as well as nausea-inducing drugs have not been used in the UK since the 1970s, though apparently they're still used in China. They were replaced in the 1980s by conversion therapy through talking. And you no longer get it on the NHS; it is mainly connected to religious organisations who want to 'pray the gay away'.

Plans are in place to ban conversion therapy altogether in the UK, as it has been in other countries. Some argue against that, saying people who want to be 'converted' to heterosexuality have a right to choose conversion therapy, and it should be made available to them as long as they consent to it, rather than be made illegal. Well, Jeremy 'consented' to his aversion therapy. When someone is vulnerable, consent can all too easily be gained through coercion.

What does Jeremy think of this argument to give people the 'choice' to be converted? You guessed it.

Fuck off.

Here is Jeremy's happy ending. Red and green house. Dog on the sofa. Pentagram hanging next to the hearth: the Stephen talisman, his most precious belonging. When he dies, he's going to have the pentagram buried with his ashes. Dry stone wall-building in beautiful places. Pints at his local. Daydreams of his beautiful boy. A reconnection with the young Jeremy. A deep understanding of what has happened to him, of what his brain has done to protect him. Forgiveness of himself.

No need or desire to forgive his parents or the Catholic Church or that Headmaster. Because why? They don't deserve it.

They can just fuck right off.

# Of Sound Mind. Mostly.

## Joyia Fitch

### Working with Clare Mackintosh

## The GP

*London, 2016*

I'm at the doctor's for a sore throat.

'What were you doing in Bali all this time?' Perhaps he can see my thousand-yard stare, maybe he's spotted my weight loss. I'm thinner, leaner; maybe weaker, maybe stronger, I can't really tell. I try not to flinch as he examines my neck glands, his fingers prodding around.

*What were you doing in Bali?* His question smudges me like an eraser, my reply tiny scuffs of rolled rubber. 'Yoga . . . this woman . . . jungle . . .' The scuffs fall across his desk and into the old black keyboard his chubby fingers tap away on.

Scuff, scuff, scuff. Tap, tap, tap.

He turns from his screen, clasps his hands and looks me in the eye. 'I think you have PTSD.' I can't run anywhere, any more.

I'm unblurred, for a moment. How someone can tell that in a ten-minute appointment, I'll never know. *Post-traumatic stress disorder* — isn't that what war-torn soldiers get?

I go to the doctor's for a sore throat. I walk out with a mental health referral.

## Being with Yoo

*Ubud, Bali, 2012*

Yoo holds her tiny hand out towards me as I hover at the edge of the circle. Seven of her followers sit under a palm umbrella, their brightly coloured yoga attire matching the sky-blaze above. I'd only been hanging around for a few weeks, my curiosity deepening as to what this mysterious Yoo was all about. Gingerly, I place my hand in Yoo's little palm and softness instantly switches to electricity – the shot surges straight up, zapping my always-and-forever shoulder tension. Zap, zap, zap. She pulls me – her grip firm – and I allow her to. I tuck in tight next to her and inhale the sweetness of her sweat.

'I can smell you,' I whisper.

'It's *soma*, the elixir of yoga.' Our deep breaths wave in and out in unison. I notice it distinctly and I'm sure she notices it too. 'Drink it up, Joy-Star.'

We lie back and Yoo's long, gorgeous, frangipani-scented black hair creeps into my dirty-blonde split-ended locks. I blink and imagine it as our interlocking nervous systems. Seeping. Spreading. Spiralling.

Together . . . Tightening.

My heart skips a breath-beat as her delicate fingers move up my spine, playing every vertebra like an instrument, checking out each note's possibility. She grunts and my whole body jerks, a neck jolt too. Puppet strings pulled for a test run.

Maybe I'll stay? Just for a while.

There's nowhere else for me to be.

The West wasn't working out for me anyway. I wasn't understanding the expectations of mortgages, full-time jobs, relationships. So, I'd wandered and wondered, looking, searching for where I might fit in, where my true place in the world might be. Belonging maybe.

'Now I *really* want to run away,' I tell her.

'Sure you do, you've been running your whole life.' We both sit up. I look into her amber eyes, but they are too bright. I look away. 'I wonder what would happen if you stopped, really stopped and looked at your programmes, your filters, your masks, your conditionings – the fake you. Your *False Identity?*'

'I don't know.' The tropical swelter sucks up the single tear rolling down my cheek.

'A *False Identity* stands between you and your fullest potential, your fullest power, your fullest you; between you and source energy. I'll reflect everything back to you, I'll be the source. I'll orchestrate it all, crystal clear.'

'Just *offer up your transparency*, speak what's true to you in the moment.' The sing-song suggestion comes from Amrita, Am for short; she is one of Yoo's most loyal followers, and the friend who introduced me to her. 'It's simple, and *stay in the gratitude*. Twelve of us are heading to the jungle with Yoo soon for a five-week Tathya. You coming?'

'Tathya?'

'The Ultimate Truth. An immersion.'

It all sounds deeper than the other cuddle-puddle, airy-fairy bullcrap I'd encountered in Ubud on my previous trips. Maybe I *could* do with getting rid of my mask and conditionings; all the shit holding me back. Is enlightenment really real? Is there something more? In *practice*, Yoo takes us through breathing exercises and sun or moon salutations with mantra where the penetrating sound of her voice tinkers around under my skin. Animal noises escape from Yoo and her followers' lips, but I try not to judge such strangeness. My patient crane pose is crap and wobbly and my tree pose falls more often than it stands straight. Sometimes I have a purple colour in my head in corpse pose but I think I'll never be able to do a perfect headstand.

'I've never seen Yoo hold her hand out to anyone like that.' Worthless folds her arms and I feel her eyes settle on me, narrowing. Yoo has gifted most of us with new names. Worthless blatantly got the weirdest one.

'I could watch Yoo and Joy-Star lying there all day.' Max, forever attending to Yoo's every need, pours her more chai. He's the only one living with Yoo; everyone else lives alone, or together in rentals across town. 'Their breath in perfect synchronicity.'

'Yes, an invisible thread is forming between us, an energetic symbiosis, of a very, very unethical love affair.' Yoo's words paint themselves over me. 'And she's an innocent – she hasn't read the books.' Everyone laughs, except me and Yoo.

It's true; I know nothing of deities or Sanskrit, but I'd be lying if I said I didn't feel special. I feel . . . I feel . . . I feel the safest I have ever been. I look down at my bronzed feet in my Havaianas flip-flops. My nails are unvarnished now, because Yoo says it's toxic – it will interfere with my awakening.

I believe her.

I believe everything.


## The Cult Specialist

*London, 2016*

I wipe my rain-sodden Doc Martens on Dr Stone's doormat which says, 'Welcome' in big red letters. I got lost at the crossroads getting off the Tube, unsure I'd ever be found. Dr Stone offers me tea, a chocolate bourbon, a custard cream. I refuse all but the tea.

'Some things I experienced were *magic*.' I bite my thumbnail and my eyes flick over the rows of academic books behind her. It's all so textbook.

She breathes in and out. It's not the first time someone has said that to her. 'The yoga and meditations can be dissociating,' she says. 'Do you feel like you space out? You could try stopping the practices for a while.' Blue ink bubbles from her biro as she draws a triangle and writes *Yoo* at the top. We analyse the layering, how money and resources go upwards, rarely downwards; how front groups hide what's really going on. I tell Dr Stone that Yoo is charismatic and smart, and that I think I still love her. I tell her I'm always spacing out.

'These leaders are psychopaths. Narcissists. They break people to control them, they're experts at word salad.' Drops of spittle land on the map of my experience. 'They have no psychological training to work with people's minds, no safe space.'

It's a bitter pill, so I choose not to swallow.

'I'm waiting to get some therapy,' I tell her. 'The doctor thinks I might have PTSD. I keep having flashbacks. I jump at the slightest thing.'

'Good idea. I know of a cult recovery group that you could go to; they meet once a month.'

'Thanks. I'll think about it.' Fuck joining another group.

'You know, cults aren't all that different from other controlling relationships. Maybe you can see some of these dynamics in your past; in people you know, perhaps. Coercive control is a crime here now.' Behind her round glasses, her eyes sparkle with a wisdom I can't refute. I'm busted. 'It'll be a while before it includes cults, though.'

I start crying and she gently pushes a box of tissues towards me. I know exactly what she's talking about; a history that made me susceptible, suggestible even. But I'm not going to talk about that. It's far too big. I watch her stir her tea. Bound to be PG Tips or Yorkshire. Reliable. Bog-standard. Boring. Her teaspoon clink, clink, clinks the flowery porcelain like a wake-up call.

'Now you can see your experience through fresh eyes. Education is the best protection.'

'I don't think it's going to be as simple as that.' I get up from the scratchy, hessian-cushioned chair. 'I might like to see you again though.'

It can't do any harm. Right?

'Of course, take your time. One day at a time. Know there is support, OK? Next time we'll talk about trauma bonds and attachment theory.'

I fold the triangle drawing and put it in my pocket.

I don't get lost at the crossroads.

Perhaps I'll be found after all.


## Shapeshifting

*Kintamani, Bali, 2012*

'Your face is huge!' I laugh. My eyes can't take it in. I shriek. I'm in my own universe. 'Your face has gone huge, Am, it's like a moon. The Moomins, a Moomin.' I'm awestruck by my vision; it's like being on drugs, but there's no drugs. Yoo is far too clean-living for that, so it must be *magic*, surely? Four months of being with Yoo and I'm here, three weeks into Tathya.

I crawl back to Yoo. The fire crackles and burns, spits red

sparks behind her. Her face morphs. It blends into a man's, a plump teenager's, a panther's before shifting, slideshow-like, into the faces of the dead people of my life. All the griefs and sorrows that follow me around are rising. I'm reliving all my regrets, all my injustices, all my fantasies, all the things I wished for but weren't true. I practise *offering up transparency*, upchucking all my unresolved everythings in colours I never knew were in me, out here in the middle of an emerald jungle nowhere.

'What do you say?' she demands.

I look into her eyes. Chocolate, milky brown, orange. Deep. I get close to her face, looking, wanting to play. I move in closer, in my head I think *play, play, play.* I get real close to her face and—

She flings me backwards. Pushes my chin back. I grab hold of her shoulders. She raises her right hand and two fingers press deep down on my throat. Her thumb, too – pressing, pressing.

I'm flat on the bamboo floor. Immobilised.

Breathe. Press. Breathe. Press. My pulse fights in my neck veins. I'm defenceless. Just a lamb.

Breathe. Press. Breathe. Press. Is it love? I barely breathe. Everyone is silent.

Yoo eases her grip and releases me.

'What do you say?' she whispers in my ear.

I gasp-breathe. 'I love you,' I stutter.

'What else?'

I gasp-breathe. 'Thank you,' I stutter.

Yoo rises and falls and I rise and fall straight into her arms.

'Energy points, *marma points*, where life energy exists, are designed to heal,' Yoo purrs. 'Or kill.'

Two fingers. Press. And thumb.

Little rattan wicker lamps, magnetising moths to their fates, light the way for Worthless to get me back to our bamboo bungalow, where I dribble and wail into the night, my neck bruises marbling into existence. Worthless already has her own neck bruises, and she doesn't leave my side. I look into her eyes, but they are all black. There are no whites to her eyes. There are no backs to her eyes. Horror.

The fat grey monkey is eating tiny bananas on our balcony at our 5 a.m. stirring. I look up and count the speckled dots of tropical mould on the ceiling as I chant 108 *So Hum*s, a mantra meaning *I am that*. I gargle with turmeric hot water, scrape my tongue, wash my eyes with rose water and give myself a warm oil massage before showering. Yoo blows her conch after leading six rounds of sun salutations at speed where we hold our breath just before cobra pose. At Tathya, none of us are calling or emailing our families or friends, none of us are logging on to Facebook – we call it FalseIDbook now. We know better, and people out there won't understand. 'They won't have the context,' Yoo says. If I hold my hand up against the white flashes of light striking through the wild, tangled green leaves, if I melt and meld to them, am I truly here? We chant into the night, offering obscurations to the fire at ceremony. All our nakedness. I hear Yoo's voice reverberating like a cymbal in my head: 'This path is not for everyone, your *False Identity* will resist its death. But you, Joy-Star, you are doing the work, you are waking up.'

Yoo kill me. Yoo free me.

## The Honorary Counselling Psychologist

*London, 2016*

'It doesn't sound like paranoia – your life really was threatened.'

I imagine Ian in his office. A computer in front of him; his notebooks and reams of emails to get through. I'm on one of the numerous telephone assessments and check-ins I've had over many, many months. It's a relief to hear his words. I don't think I'm paranoid either, but I can't be sure.

'There's the death of myself,' I try to explain. 'Within myself, my *False Identity* death.' I pull my coat tighter around me, protecting me from the November chill. 'And then there are the death threats, if I ever go back there.' I pick a flake of green paint off the poles of the bandstand in Ruskin Park where I'm sheltering from the downpour, my hands slightly quivering. Pick, pick, pick. My life.

'The "splits" you speak of,' Ian says. 'Your "False Identity" death. They were most likely stress-induced psychotic episodes. And the shakes are your nervous system's attempt to regulate itself in such a long-sustained trauma. In terms of treatment, Eye Movement Desensitisation and Reprocessing might not be sensible, as you were experiencing trance states and EMDR might trigger them.'

Trance states?

But *magic*. But *kundalini awakening*. But *shakti*. But *tantra*. But *vishuddhi chakra*. But *crown opening* . . .

But . . . it could be true, what Ian says. The body did keep the score after all.

'I must ask you. Are you thinking of hurting yourself?'

'No.'

'That's good.'

'Do you know when I might be able to see someone?'

'I'm so sorry the waiting list is so long. I can put you in touch with our community counselling. You can talk some things through with a trainee psychologist. It won't be as structured as the trauma-focused CBT, but it might be helpful?'

'Yes, please do.'
I need all the help I can get.


## The Cutting

*Ubud, Bali, 2012*

I cut. I cut five times. I don't know why I am cutting five times instead of once. I can't find the reason for that. I don't know what to do, so I cut. I cut five times. It's easy. I love the feeling, the sensation. It doesn't hurt. It takes me out of my stuck-in-sensitivity spin-out, where lines fail to draw themselves where my body ends, and the strangling air begins. This will bring me back. I love the blood run. The moment I slice, it looks like nothing is happening; a gap and then, then the opening, the release, the drip around. It varies – it might be little blood bubbles first, or it might be a straight gash rising. Depends on how deep I go on each slice. When hard meets soft, where red glistens like toffee-apple trickle on the canvas of electric-green rice field. An after-sting sensation, buzzing. The patch-up and a lingering sting, a fragility. I don't know why I cut five times instead of once. I can't find the reason for that.

It's around Christmas, but it's never winter here. Dreams. Tears. I hear Yoo in me and hear Yoo's voice in the in-between, a promise to chase. Physically, I *could* leave. But my mind cannot. And so I just lie here, me and my *False Identity* that refuses to die, alone apart from when Am brings me homemade kitcheree and mango chutney. A jar of chai spice blend, too. I stroke the plasticky dark green ribbon tied awkwardly around the lid.

'A Christmas present from Yoo,' she says.

# The Trainee Counselling Psychologist

*London, 2017*

'What a fucking bitch.' 'Total mind-fuck.' The favourites of my phrases, tumbling multiple times from my mouth during our session.

Paul's are more measured. 'A lot to unpack.' 'Watchful waiting.' He diligently takes notes. What's he writing that could be so interesting?

'I'm so angry.' I catch my flushed face reflected in the window of the small box room we're in. I'm roasting. Distant sirens scream, probably from St Tommy's. I imagine joining in with them.

'You have every right to be.'

Helping Paul get his training hours on his journey of helping people makes me feel better about being fucked up. The prickle behind my nose paves the way for what's always there: splashes of sad, falling unresisted onto my tracksuit bottoms. Paul lets me cry. He's just there. When I stop, we challenge which patterns to break.

'If you're still following a similar diet to when you were in Bali, you might want to eat some meat. Heavier, grounding food.'

'Are you crazy?' I laugh. 'I'm never going to eat meat, but I *might* start eating a bit of fish again. Besides, kitcheree *is* grounding.'

I wander the streets of London after our session, crossing Waterloo Bridge in springtime. Flowers are blooming, especially the ones in Victoria Embankment Gardens. Bright purple and fuchsia pink tulips illuminate me from the inside, tempering the residue rush of rage, banishing the waterfalled tears. Perhaps there is an incoming fresh, assured scent of hope.

And, only, maybe, a sweet, faint trace of frangipani.

the split

*Ubud, Bali, 2013*

\*Happy\*Fucking\*New\*Year\*
split no sleep
i will not let you sleep
i will

p ------ >    i   < ------    n   ------ >    g   < --------

your mind

         —       from

                                      right

             to

left

there's two parts

                               two parts

cut through the

             m
             i
             d
             d
             l
             e

flopped

             either

                                 side

             sp / l / it

                         my *False Identity*
             my *False Identity*, my *False ID* goblin runs away

                    s                           s
               m                    k
                    i          r
                              thinks – ha ha, i've got you
                              it demands, persists, drains


                              DON'T DO IT Worthless
~~DON'T~~ DO IT Worthless                    you are worthy
                         it's going to be so painful for you
                            you are so well constructed
                               it's going to be so painful
                     my *False ID* is desperate to save you
                                 it's its d y i n g wish
          it wants to keep all the *False ID*s on the same team
                              DON'T DO IT Amrita
                                 i see you in me
                         you don't know what's there yet
                            there's so much in you Am


~~DON'T~~ DO IT Am


                                        people don't know
                                           i didn't know
                                         i was so ignorant


                                    i didn't know what the *sp*
                    *l*
*it* was

                                    i didn't know what this was
                                        it seems like words
                                           just something
              this is the most painful thing i have ever experienced

                                    i Am wARniNg yOu
                                     it is grip-fast
                                        steadfast
                                 & i know it's not over
                                it's going to turn WiLdeR

          i have not gotten real until now
          what a faker
          i hate Yoo
          Yoo are crushing me


## The Cult Recovery and Support Group

*London, 2017*

I walk into the hotel conference room in Marylebone and instantly want to leave.

I don't, because a guy in his early twenties with mild acne has made me a green tea from the urn. There are three purple-rinse haired ladies whose children are all in the same "religion", another who's leaving a political organization, and someone who was in a multi-level marketing company. There's also a couple of people from spiritual groups not too dissimilar to mine.

'Do you have family here?' one of the purple-rinse haired mums asks. 'Are you working?'

'Yes.' I shuffle in my faux-pine chair. 'I'm back and functioning . . . kind of well, I think. I mean . . . I'm still tired all the time.'

'It was only three years, I'm sure you'll do just fine.' Her smile is warm, her pale grey eyes a little sad. 'Your mother must be so relieved you came back.'

She's right, my mum is relieved. There's support everywhere I turn. There's probably a recovery group for everything. And three years isn't a lifetime.

116

Isn't it so strange? Isn't it so strange the things that people believe?

split / break

*Ubud, Bali, 2013*

                                        ~~no.~~ don't stay there
come back

                                        are you fucking stupid?
my head is in so much pain

                                        t~e~r~r~o~r
                                        i can't get out
                                        my forehead burns red
                            my *False ID* will not let me look at
the other side
i've fucked it up

                                        i don't know who i am
                        depersonalisation is a mental disorder
my *False ID* has my gratitude in its gnashers

                                            gnawing
                                    ~~no, no~~ gratitude
                                        that kills me

that makes the real stronger
the truth stronger

                    split / knife

Am asks me, what's

                                        the other side?

it's Yoo
e v e r y t h i n g is Yoo

Y o o  i s  everything
true. real
i feel Yoor presence
Yoo have filled me up
i stretch my head back                              n
Yoo loves me so much               e               d
my neck                    b                            s
                                                              all
                                      the
                        way
          k      c      a      b


Yoo have already won
i am calm
peace

                                        for a moment


                    split / pop


              my *False ID* wants to keep me away from Yoo
                              don't see Yoo
~~DON'T~~ SEE YOO

                                        she is killing me
                                           look at you
                                        you are a mess
                        ~~end it~~ now tell Yoo to STOP
                                   can't go any further now
                                          got to go away
                                               enough
                                        i've fucked it up
                              & it's never going to end
              are you kidding me?


                              118

you really think i am going to let you sit in the

A*W*E

that weakens me

& **strengthens** you

don't you know how **strong** i am?
Ha ha. Yoo've got to be kidding
i'm too smart & shift able
forget it
Max, how  l  o  n  g  does this fucking last?
i'm dying
i'm shrinking . . .

Family

*Surrey, 2017*

I pour gravy on my nut roast. Broccoli. My too-cute niece's and nephews' squeals of delight drown out the *Antiques Roadshow* theme tune. I watch them roll their Brussels sprouts in ketchup. Sticky fingers. Cauliflower.

'Another spud, Jo-Jo?'

'Go on then, Papa.'

'I'm happy you're home,' says my mum.

I close my eyes, take a deep breath. 'Me too.' Just my own breath now.

Recovery is a fucking minefield.

But here is love.

Apple crumble and custard.

119

# A Sound Mind

*Ubud, Bali, 2013*

'Blood-letting is a medical procedure to cure disease, *dis-ease*.' Yoo's voice scrapes like a shard of glass across the soft, turned-inside-out creases of my brain. 'Tribal, branding, offering, sacrifice. You can get fruit from this if you choose the blessing, not the curse.'

I sit blankly. My denim shorts are almost falling off me. I'm disguised as a girl. Purifying. Unsure of who or what is me and who or what is masquerading as me. My *False ID*. The long table stretches to the side of me and Worthless. Am and Max's faces blur into a single sorrowful one. I breathe deeply, but my face feels like it's slipping in fragments. Parts falling off.

'I feel like balancing somehow, but either side is quicksand, it's fucking dangerous.' I stuff a chapati into my mouth, when all I really want to do is lick the ghee off it. 'On my scooter, I feel like I'm flying.'

'It must be what Joy-Star needs on a soul level.' Am scratches the tiny red spots beneath the band of bay leaves tied around her forehead, an attempt to bring down her constant feverish headaches. She looks like Pocahontas.

'You shouldn't be riding your scooter.' Yoo takes a meticulously measured sip of chai. 'Run. Run, slowly. And a sound mind is essential.'

'Worthless told me Yoo said I didn't have one.' A quiver of shame in my voice.

'Let's look at this.' Her tiny fingers tap her glass mug. 'Bring it to the front. A sound mind . . . a sound mind is in the one who has absolute faith in my love for them, that they know without a shadow of doubt that they are absolutely loved. The question has always been whether you can sit in the heart of

120

the paradox.' She places her hand on her heart, her deliverance settling onto the sweaty skins of her audience, reaching into their bodies, as it does into mine. 'Whether you can meet me where I am at. Any of you?'

Nobody says anything. Deafening silence.

Maybe we are all the wise fools. My brow furrows, my eyes squint.

Hang on.

That's not what a sound mind is.


## The Friend

*London, 2017*

'You seemed completely out of it. Inaccessible.' James sips his Malbec. Brown curls cover the ears he's always been self-conscious about. 'Of course, we talked about what to do.' We're in our old haunt from our acting days on Drury Lane. Fairy lights twinkle on our wine glasses, mirroring the sparkle of the West End's promising stardust.

'You didn't *actually* do anything, though, did you?' I laugh, but I'm only half joking.

'It was tricky. I researched. We didn't want to push you further away. I read if you confront a cult member it's a no win.'

'I probably would have been even more loyal to her.'

'We just tried to keep communication open with you, even when you were defensive.'

'I'm sorry.' The oaky Malbec sticks like chocolate in my throat. 'I wasn't well.'

'I know. You're never going back, are you?'

'I don't think so. I keep getting triggered when I get an email from someone connected or see an online exposé of another cult.'

'So don't look at it. You've got a million other things you're into, all the old things you love. Focus on them again.'

I do.


## I Got Out

*Ubud, Bali and everywhere else*

Yoo leisurely picks her front teeth with a toothpick, until she draws it out of her mouth and angles it towards me. 'Sign my waiver and NDA.'

'No.' My eyes close in on the minuscule pale tip of the toothpick. Yoo's face blurs and smudges behind it, her milky-pink silk kaftan almost transparent.

I blink away, look down at my cuts and lightly trace one of them with my finger. It's the first day I've been able to take the plasters off, and the dirt-cream sticky residue still grazes my skin. I see Yoo's hand shaking under the table, hidden from the restaurant staff who always give us the side-eye.

Am softly taps the waiver and NDA documents with a biro. Tap, tap, tap. I avoid eye contact with her but imagine smashing her Ray-Ban sunglasses down off her head and into her smug eyeballs. I can feel Max staring at me, Worthless too. Is Yoo shitting herself? I'm shitting myself. I'm not the first to say I'm going to jump off a bridge.

'My *False ID* will not sign anything.' My toes scrunch up in my scuffed Havaianas.

'You've curdled. You can go, Joy-Star. Sorry, *Joyia*.' A needle-scrape to my eardrums. 'The petals will fall. It's nature's way. New circle, new flower. That's right, run away.'

I feel myself dropping, floating. I want to catch myself in petal form as I fall, and press myself inside a book for safekeeping. But I do not need to keep or cling to her. She is in me, my petal of me. I put a crisp, pink 100-rupiah note on the table. I'm done with the diet of egg-white omelette, dal and chai. I'd kill for a coffee or a glass of wine.

I click the clasp on my musty-smelling scooter helmet and scoop up my keys. 'Bye.' I wish I had the guts to say *fuck off*.

'So be it.' Her fingers flick, the jitterbug still undercurrenting them. My ribs react, as though she has cast magical hundreds and thousands inside me. A kind of pain and a kind of freedom strikes through me. Spiced smoke from the incense sticks that line the streets whorls around me as I scooter off up Jalan Hanoman. Just like that.

But I don't leave 'just like that'. Leaving a dynamic like this rarely happens in a heartbeat, nor is it often just a one-time leaving. I run as far as I can, to Thailand, to London, to South Korea to teach English, before eventually returning to Yoo, unable to sleep her off, shake her off. My head *splits* again, and Yoo calls this my *crown opening*. It isn't as bad as the other time and I don't cut myself again, but the dead people of my life visit me again, surge through me, snap me in half. I run, I run again, I run to Nepal.

A mango smoothie sherbets my tongue in a little café on a dusty side street in Pokhara. My hands shake as I google *Cult Specialist London* on intermittent internet. *Click*. A woman who has written books about it. *Click*. An email address. *Click*. Everything begins to click, click, click.

*I think I've just left a cult*, I type.

*Click*.

# The High-Intensity Cognitive Behavioural Therapist

*London, 2017*

'How can we continue a safe space for you moving forward?' Even with her fancy title, in skinny jeans and ballet pumps, Kate doesn't seem all that much older than me. 'Trauma can make you feel like you're back there. Emotions and fears flood back.' She's always asking me what I think. 'How do you think you're going to manage that?'

'I don't know.'

'Imagery that involves a safe, protective space might work. You're creative, can you think of a safe space? I know we aren't in the most inspiring of rooms.'

I look around at the dull cream walls laden with remnants of dried Blu Tack. Beams of late autumnal sepia stream through the window, falling across filing cabinets and cardboard folders in precarious piles.

'A shield or a bubble. Or both.'

'Can you imagine them?'

'The bubble is transparent, it can move in and out and allow or not allow. The shield is big, dark blue and metal. There's a circle and I'm inside holding the shield. I know what's inside is worth protecting, I know it's worthy.'

'What do you think keeps the bubble strong?' Kate smiles.

'Being centred in my own power. Knowing I've got the control stick, that I can turn away and that's OK. Managing my own space. Boundaries. Respect.'

I truly own these words. I sound like me.

'Hold that image. I want you to think if there is any trigger that just' – she clicks her fingers *left, right, left, right* – 'takes you back to where you were again. What will bring this image of this bubble and this shield, so you can start to feel it?'

'Standing in a strong stance, my feet rooted.'

'OK. Quite often with trauma, triggers can happen out of the blue. You can access this image of you being in this protective bubble and being strong, the soles of your feet on the floor. Access to this safe place is in your toolbox. A safe place isn't just where you go and hide. Or are protected. It's also where you stand up and it's almost like: I'm ready for this.'

My Doc Martens press into the weird, thin blue carpet, the kind of carpet that maybe isn't even carpet at all. 'I've got my shield.' I tell her. 'My conviction.'

'Yes, being assertive. Following your own beliefs rather than other people's, or hiding away.'

I didn't trust my own judgement for so long.

I let other people decide what was best for me.

Not any more.


## Afterwards

I want to write that I'm fully recovered! I'm through the other side! I'm healed! I'm totally over it! I've moved on! I have it all figured out!

But that wouldn't be true.

The truth is, it took years to leave, and I didn't do it alone; four other brave ones left with me. Together we worked it out as we worked ourselves out of Yoo's control. We started talking about what had happened to us, and in telling our stories, we started to heal. We helped each other see with fresh eyes, the *fresh eyes* Dr Stone was talking about. But it all took time. Lots of time. I couldn't have left without their support.

Though I am better than before, so much better, I do still get triggered every now and then, but it doesn't scare me as much as it used to. It doesn't own me. I realise I can still be affected by my experience from time to time, but not defined by it. I don't get the shakes like I used to. I haven't seen faces shapeshift again, I haven't seen eyes with no backs to them and I haven't been visited by the dead people of my life. I haven't seen anyone's head expand to five times its regular size. I'm a healthy weight with a buffer to protect my nervous system. I drink wine more than I probably should. Coffee, too. I'm partial to a bit of sugar.

In 2018, I dusted off my blush-red Osprey backpack with the side zips and adventured through north Thailand and south India. I found my own connection to yoga, meditation, ayurveda and ritual. It certainly is magic when it isn't being manipulated for mind-fuckery. I began to truly feel freer than ever before; I'd found my way home, my home within me.

I came to understand that Yoo was shaped by the traumas and griefs of her past. She doesn't think what she's doing is wrong – I saw she knew no other way. When I think of her in that way, I can feel a softness. Her history doesn't excuse her actions but it's important to acknowledge it. Part of me still loves her, misses her. People might think I'm still under the spell. I am a bit. Perhaps. In many ways, she *was* there for me. The tenderest of moments, moments I haven't written about here, have etched themselves and tightly knotted themselves into my heart. The love was there, it was real.

A version of it.

It's complicated.

But I can also protect myself. I have no regrets, but maybe I can only say that because I survived to tell the tale. It could easily have been different. I miss Am, Worthless, Max and a few of the others too. Sometimes I wonder how they are, where they are, but it scares me to try to find out.

My mind loops back from time to time, wonders what was right or wrong. Ponders the nuances of love, magic; logic, reason. But I realise that my *False Identity* isn't false at all. It's a part of me, an essence of me. I need it.

And maybe that's it: finding a way to understand, not a quest for absolute recovery. Do you ever recover from life?

Would I seek help and support again? Absolutely, of course.

Am I of sound mind?

Mostly. It's a life's work.

I pick up the pieces of paper, all the notes along the way I have made to set free this story. The brainstorming, the memories, the creases embedded in A4 sheets folded into sixteen possible sections; the cross-outs and the leave-ins of all the people, the dates, the moments; red pen marked up against green pen; places visited on this plane and otherwise. I rub out my scrawlings over and over, making sense of it all again and again, and I watch as the faint cursive lines lift themselves up off the pages. I blow the tiny scuffs away and they dash like jumping beans, dropping, falling. Pieces of me. The parts that make up everything that happened to me.

I had to run away to truly run towards. Towards a new me.

A me that better knows my own mind.

A me that loves me.

A me that trusts me.

# A Pair of Slippers:

## It's easier to put on a pair of slippers than to carpet the whole world

### Sarah

### As told to Joanna Cannon

For as long as I can remember, everything I have done, everything I have said, what I was and am, and will be, has all been decided for me. I have no control over it, no choice in the matter. Because everything I did and everything I thought, everything I *was*, had to first pass through a filter. A filter I have lived with since I was a child.

I feel sick.

It was there when I opened my eyes.

I feel sick.

I would wake in the night and know it was because I needed to be sick. That's what bodies do – they wake up in the middle of the night if something is wrong. And mine was waking up because the worst thing in the world was about to happen. It didn't happen, but that didn't prove that it wouldn't or that it couldn't, or that it won't happen next time.

I feel sick.

What should I have for breakfast? Should I even eat breakfast or am I mistaking nausea for hunger? Perhaps I shouldn't eat anything until I'm sure. Or maybe it's better not to eat at all, because that would be much safer. Wouldn't it?

I feel sick.

The thought was a constant companion. I was in perpetual terror. It was with me every waking hour, and it was so loud it sometimes woke me from my sleep. Because I have emetophobia (the medical term for fear of vomiting) and emet (as it's known by those who live with it) ensures every single thought, feeling, emotion and movement needs to pass through the phobia before it can exist separately. I could look at a flower, and I could see it and appreciate its beauty, but it existed only after passing through some kind of thought, feeling or twinge relating to vomit. In those usually blissful moments before being fully awake, those fractions of seconds when you just start to realise you're no longer unconscious but not yet sure exactly where you are or what life is, emetophobia would blare out its favourite anthem: 'I FEEL SICK'. I wouldn't even have a chance to process it before emetophobia staked its claim on my mind : yes. YES. YES. And so, in the first thirty seconds of my waking hours I would already have started experiencing a panic attack. Of course, panic like this works in perfect harmony with insomnia and bad sleeping, so I had little chance to escape its entrapments.

Emetophobia has coloured and flavoured everything I have interacted with, both internally and externally, and it's woven into my mind, burrowed so deep into who I am, that I can no longer separate it from myself. It's part of me. It *is* me. I can't tell you why it exists, or explain why I am beholden to it, but

I can tell you when it first appeared, when my life became controlled and dictated by a single thought.

I was thirteen. My mum put a plate of food in front of me. Something I ate regularly; something I usually enjoyed, even. I can't say what the food was, because the words alone frighten and repulse me, even now. But I remember the smell and the texture. I remember staring into this plate of food and experiencing a sudden, visceral reaction to it, being engulfed by a terror so great and so overwhelming, I couldn't even recognise it for what it was: a panic attack. If you have never experienced a panic attack, the idea of one won't make sense to you, however hard people try to describe it. I felt like I was dying, wanted to die and already dead, all at the same time. To a thirteen-year-old, it was terrifying. A sudden wave of dread and terror came over me which was so great, I was no longer able to see the room around me, to feel the weight of my body on the chair, to hear my mum's voice. I was unable to move, to think, to smell, to hear, to see, to respond. I was made of nothing but fear and I didn't know why.

I remember being utterly dazed by this bodily response to something I ate frequently, to the process of eating which I usually relished, but once that response arrived in my life, it refused to leave. Even when I wasn't experiencing panic, the idea of it was there, and the anticipation of having another attack, the burden of carrying all that fear around with me, became too much. For six years, I would experience around ten panic attacks a day. During my panic attacks, I would space out and dissociate from reality, becoming totally unaware of my surroundings. They are so insular, panic attacks, so utterly internalised. To anyone else I probably just looked like I'd zoned out, but in actual fact I was incredibly zoned in – into my stomach, any slight twinge I felt or imagined, zoned into the repetitive thoughts, of knowing the worst thing in the world was happening or about to happen. The thing that would end all things.

It took me a while before I was able to express in words how bad things were, how much I was struggling to get through each day, because even though I was only a teenager, I wasn't just carrying around a fear of being sick, I was carrying around so many other things as well. I don't recall coming across the term emetophobia, but as a child, I do remember looking up obsessive–compulsive disorder and finding a checklist where I was able to tick off almost every box. OCD was something I'd experienced for much, much longer than emet. Its origins are fuzzy but it began around the age of seven, with facial tics and compulsive routines, superstitious thinking and what's known as Pure O – intrusive thoughts of severe danger and harm. Everything I saw on the news was going to happen to me or someone I loved. It wasn't a question of *if*, it was a question of *when*. I looked at everyone with suspicion, a potential threat. A minute of not knowing where my mum was would send me into a breakdown – I knew she was dead. She was not, of course, dead, but my brain forced me into thinking the worst with such surety that logic and reason never even got a chance to make an appearance.

By the time emetophobia added itself to the list, I had already spent most of my younger years in a state of severe anxiety. Most people remember their childhood as a series of happy events. Holidays, birthday parties, days out with their families. My memories of childhood are restricted only to what I felt internally, the constant stream of worries and the compulsions I carried out to allay them. I didn't really link emetophobia to these symptoms until a few years in, seeing it as something in and of itself that had taken over my entire system of functioning, but emetophobia is a form of OCD (perhaps it's also a front for lots of other things, which is a question I've not yet found the answer to). The fear of something happening causes you to come up with rituals, called compulsions (the 'C' of OCD) that in the short term soothe the obsession, but in the long term amplify it. Physically, my main compulsion was – and still is – excessive hand-washing. In my worst times, I would undertake my hand-washing ritual every twenty minutes. Mainly, though, my compulsions were internal, indiscernible to others. Essentially, by constantly holding on to the thought that I would be sick, I would be able to prevent myself from being sick. It was absolutely crucial to hold on to that anxiety in order to keep myself safe. If a moment went by where I wasn't thinking about vomiting, then I would surely commit some terrible action that would lead to it happening. The phobia became both my captor and my saviour.

I was referred to CAMHS – Child and Adolescent Mental Health Services – when I was fourteen, and I started seeing a therapist once a week. The only appointment they had available was in the middle of the day, meaning I had to skip school. I would leave school alone, and return alone afterwards. NHS mental health waiting lists are long, so at the time I felt very lucky to be given that slot, but walking into a hospital as someone with emetophobia is a challenging experience. The first problem presented itself at the door. I, an emetophobe with severe germ and health OCD, had to walk through a hospital, the most germ-ridden place imaginable to my young mind, in order to receive treatment. No one met me at the entrance or helped me make my way to the CAMHS department. Every week I would fill with panic, hold my breath, hand sanitiser grasped firmly in my fist, and walk in. I would have to wait for someone else to walk down the corridor to open the multiple doors because I was too terrified to touch them. I was traumatised before my appointment even began.

In the CAMHS waiting room, I would sit and look around at all the other sick young people, seeing those much more visibly ill than I was. Teenagers so thin they looked barely more than skeletons, adolescents with thick welts down their arms, self-harm marks that made you want to weep just looking at them. Every time I walked into that waiting room, appearing to the world as relatively normal, I questioned my right to be there at all. Anxiety does that to you. It not only makes your thoughts tangled and uncertain, it makes you doubt whether you are even worthy of the help you need to untangle them. I also far too frequently saw people I knew, more than once having to hide outside the waiting room until they were ushered into an office before I could return. I was terrified of being seen there. I was not outwardly mentally unwell, despite how intensely my internal world was dominated by the illness, and I didn't tell people that I was in therapy. To this day, very few people in my life know the extent of my illness, even as I've become more open to sharing my experiences. As a young teen, I barely understood what I was going through myself, let alone how to begin to explain it to someone else.

CAMHS should have been the place where I learned to do that, but it was not a good experience for me. The NHS is a wonderful thing and I cherish it deeply, but psychiatric systems are not built on a basis of care and support. They are about enforcement – of medication, treatment, involuntarily sectioning – of curing something inherently bad for society rather than treating a human being who needs help. I was traumatised by CAMHS, and I know so many others with similar experiences. I was frequently passed between different therapists, each of whom referred me onwards in exasperation and exhaustion at not being able to really understand what I was going through and what care I needed. I received so many different types of therapy: CBT (cognitive behavioural therapy), EMDR (eye movement desensitisation and reprocessing therapy), hypnotherapy, psychodynamic education, psychotherapy and regular counselling. Emetophobia simply didn't fall neatly into any one diagnosis. It was a few different types of OCD mixed with some generalised anxiety disorder, but I was also struggling to eat and so they became side-tracked and marked me as having an eating disorder for a while, until I angrily convinced them they were very far off the mark. Someone with emet doesn't lose weight because they are focused on losing weight. They lose weight because, in the mind of an emetophobe, if you don't eat, you can't be sick. As time went on, I also became quite seriously depressed, perhaps unsurprisingly, but this got so bad that they were forced to change my care priorities to focus on the depression, and the emetophobia was discarded, even though it had gone nowhere. The whole time I was under CAMHS I felt that they simply didn't know what to do with me. More than this, though, I was dealt with as a problem, a burden they couldn't shift. I was untreatable, exhausting, difficult.

The situation was compounded by the fact that I was unwilling to get better. This is a difficult and painful truth of which I was deeply ashamed. My understanding, though, is that this is not uncommon. When you have a fear of something, you do things that you believe will keep you safe. Being better means letting go of those things, risking not feeling safe, and that is far more terrifying than any other aspect of the whole experience. I think people understand it better in something like anorexia. An anorexic is terrified of putting on weight, so if getting better is framed as being able to eat again, an anorexic mind will not want to get better, because all those safety measures will be removed. It was the same for me, and it took me a long time before I was ready to engage in therapy, to let go of keeping safe, and begin the process of recovery. Unfortunately, though, my illusion that CAMHS was there to help me was shattered when, about four years into my treatment, they suggested I try exposure therapy.

It will be hard to imagine for those who have not experienced it what it felt like when it was suggested, in all seriousness, after I'd spent four years explaining how my life, my soul, my entire being were dominated by a fear of throwing up, that the best solution would be to induce me to vomit. To take a medication that would make me throw up. To do the thing that I was so scared of. I'd rather have died. And that's how serious emetophobia was to me for so long – I would rather have died than throw up. I was also frightened, now, by the very people who were supposedly meant to reduce my fear. I worried they would force this therapy on me. That they would section me for it and make it a legal requirement, or that they'd pin me down and force the medication on me. This is not dramatic: it is wholly precedented. It's what happens in psychiatric wards across the country, and across the world. I was not naive to this, and I was absolutely terrified.

It was at that point that I lost all faith in CAMHS. It was an enraging, confusing, overwhelming, terrifying and sad moment for me, amidst a life already engulfed in such intense emotions. I felt let down by the only people who I thought would ever be able to help me. It's also important to point out that there seems to be little evidence of exposure therapy working at all, especially for something like emetophobia. After I left CAMHS I actually did throw up – on two occasions, in fact. Once, on the evening of my eighteenth birthday: I had felt unwell all evening, but it had felt like a panic attack that simply wouldn't subside. I threw up three times, and I instantly felt joyful and excited. *It had happened! I had done it!* And I was . . . fine?! I sent selfies to the one friend who knew I had it, grinning at this miracle of all miracles.

I spent the next few weeks floating, feeling light, free, unchained. But less than a month later I was in a situation where there were people around me saying they felt unwell, and in mere minutes all the old panic, the extreme flight response, the intensely powerful urge to run away overcame me. And indeed, I left that situation early, unable to be around those people any longer. I was ashamed, embarrassed by myself, devastated at the speed with which this disease seemed to have returned and the depths of my being into which it had reached. After the second bout of sickness, I had less hope that it was the cure I had been waiting for. And indeed, I was correct. If actually doing the thing didn't stop me being so terrified of it, I really felt at a loss as to how I would ever understand and recover.

Now, however, in my late twenties, I am remarkably freer of the chains of emetophobia than I ever thought possible. The process of recovery remains ongoing, but I'm privileged to have been able to pay for therapy that has been more effective. Very few people have this option. Along the way, I've also had further damaging private therapy experiences – it has not been a simple ride. It has taken me many years to find the right person, the right medication, to be in the right circumstances physically, emotionally and financially to be able to confront my mental health. For many years, this was simply not the case, and for countless others, it might never be. I feel lucky that I got there eventually, but I also recognise the impact of the trauma created by the systems available. My understanding now is that I experienced this intense phobia that centred around vomiting but it almost certainly had much deeper, more complex and nuanced roots that I am still, to this day, trying to work out.

I was asked recently, if I could go back in time, would I have emetophobia all over again? Would I keep the emetophobia, and therefore keep who I am today? And the answer is absolutely not. If I could have grown up without it, I would have taken that option in a heartbeat. There are no 'positives' of emetophobia. My story is not one of hope, it is a story of horrific internal difficulties that, over years, have lessened their grip on me. Through a mix of privilege and luck, I was able to quieten it, reduce its power, but I have never been able to let it go completely. I'm not sure I ever will. It is a terrible affliction and I wish I didn't have it, but I *can* also recognise the values it has instilled in me. I have developed a deep sense of empathy that nothing else has managed to provoke in quite the same way. I understand when someone says they *can't* do something. Not that they don't want to, or they're too lazy, tired or uninterested, but they are actually paralysed by some internal pull. I understand that pull because I have lived it. I understand what it means to simply not be able to do something that is seemingly so simple for others. I know what it feels like to be limited, constrained, out of control and totally controlled all at the same time, and it has helped me be kinder, softer and more understanding towards both loved ones and strangers.

During the worst years of my emetophobia, I didn't really feel like there was any other element to my personality. Despite almost nobody around me knowing that I had it, to me it was all I was. On top of emetophobia, over the years I have acquired multiple other diagnoses, difficulties and obsessions, and all of them together combine to make me who I am. To this day I don't know which parts of my personality are actually me, which are emetophobia or OCD, or which are a combination. Whilst mental illness is largely invisible, living with chronic anxiety catches up with you physically, and will eventually affect your appearance, your posture, the way you speak and dress, and of course, the way you behave.

I never drank alcohol for obvious reasons, and yet was able to go clubbing at university like all my peers. To outsiders, I probably came across as quite unusual, perhaps unique – not many people can go clubbing sober and dance on tables like I did, or actually enjoy – yes, enjoy – the night. I never revealed the real reason I didn't drink; I simply said it wasn't for me. At some point, that seemed to melt into truth. It's almost impossible to know whether I would ever have started drinking without it. I have never had a desire to drink or be drunk, and not just because it can make you sick. The idea of losing control like that has never enticed me. I'm an extremely controlled person – having had OCD since childhood and then a range of other anxiety problems including emetophobia, this is no surprise. But I wonder about other parts of my personality that may have benefitted from the social element of drinking, from not being the odd one out, from losing my inhibitions like everyone else. I'll never know.

Emetophobia dictated every single thought, action, feeling, decision, like and dislike. It decided who I could be around, or whether I could even be around anyone. It dictated where I could sit on a bus, and indeed if I could get on the bus at all; whether I could go somewhere and where that would be, how I could get there, how long I could stay, what I could or couldn't do when I got there – the list goes on. At college, if I knew someone in one of my classes was ill, I simply wouldn't go to that class. I couldn't be around them. If I had to be in the same room as someone who I knew was sick, I would sit as far away from them as possible, holding my breath for long periods of time, washing my hands even more frequently, running out of the room to get away as soon as possible. I remember some days not knowing where to be, as there were multiple people around me claiming to feel unwell. That person was in that classroom, so that was out of bounds. Someone else in the library rendered that location unusable, the dining room was impossible, so full of potentially sick people. I would wander around, perhaps finding an empty table in a study area of a corridor or heading outside into the glory of the fresh air.

I learned to live with my emetophobia, letting it control me and my life, my decisions, my wants and needs, and I somehow managed to still do well at school, have friends, good family relationships and enjoy extra-curricular activities. Even to me this is hard to get my head round. The way I conceptualise it now is that although I was entirely controlled by emetophobia, I was never *completely* debilitated by it. I was, to all intents and purposes, a functioning emetophobic, just like you have functioning alcoholics.

But although being able to function as an emetophobic is a strength, it has also been one of my greatest barriers to recovery. It allowed me to settle for a standard of living that I had decided was sufficient. I was unbelievably ill, but I could go through the motions of the day. Just because those motions filled me with a terror unlike anything I have ever felt, and so constantly and deeply, this didn't undermine the fact that I could, still, get through a day. I spent a lot of time researching mental illness and knew that I was not one of the worst, not by far. I had the ability to get out of bed, even if the process of doing so was so terrifying that I was exhausted before I'd even made it downstairs for breakfast. I could go to school, even if I was only focused for 50 per cent of my lessons, the other 50 per cent, or often more, spent in an internal haze of panic attacks. I had friends who were sectioned and ended up in inpatient units – I was ill but I wasn't *that* ill. I was, however, a shell of the child and teenager I could have been; a watered-down version who battled this evil power every moment of every day.

Now, for many reasons, it makes the most sense for me to work for myself. It gives me the freedom to work around my mental health when I need to, though this is not the only motivating factor (let's just say that authority and I have a complicated relationship). I remain incredibly close to my family, whose support, love and care for me throughout my worst – and best – has never wavered. My mum especially has been, at times, the only light I could see in a dark world. Like she did in my teens, she still stays on the phone with me for hours during panic attacks and constantly reminds me of my progress. Until my mid-twenties I didn't tell even my best friends about my mental health. It's an ongoing internal struggle that I still work through in therapy, but the friends I have told have been, for the most part, pretty incredible too. I am able to do so many of the things I never thought I would be able to do – travel, move out of home, live abroad, make a living. None of this means that there aren't difficult, challenging times, days overtaken by anxiety, by depression, days that feel impossible to live through.

I find it much easier to acknowledge that I may always have these moments, but that I am also able to feel joy, peace, happiness and love. And this feeling can co-exist with my feeling of sadness for the child that I was, for the child I could have been, for the adult I might have become without this illness.

Whilst in many ways it doesn't really matter, this also casts a much greater question over my existence: who am I? Do I get to exist outside of my mental illness, or has that entirely shaped who I am? Is that what personality is anyway: a shaping of oneself due to internal machinations which include mental health? Another fundamental reason I found the idea of recovery from emetophobia so difficult at first was because I didn't know who I would be without it. Despite the misery, pain, destruction and harm it caused me, it was so constant, so fundamental to my being, that I couldn't imagine a me without it. I still don't know how much of me is me and how much is *it*, but now the worst of it has subsided, I know that I am so very much more than my illness.

# All We Have Is Us

## Sanmeet Kaur

### As told to Selali Fiamanya

*'Can someone bring in some toothbrushes?'*
  *'Also, some spare towels would be really helpful!'*
I'd woken and checked my phone before doing much else
and I didn't know why my colleagues were asking for household
items on the office group chat until I turned on the news, and
it became dangerously clear: Grenfell was burning.

It was June 2017 and I worked for a small education charity
based in a church opposite the tower. That morning I took my
usual bus from my family home in Fulham, then hopped on the
Hammersmith and City Line. The ordinarily rowdy commute felt
eerily quiet, and I traded my book for Twitter, scouring for updates
as they unfolded. The walls outside Latimer Road tube station
were already plastered with 'missing' posters. I saw the faces of
students who were linked to our charity – twelve-year-olds and
five-year-olds who we had helped in after-school homework clubs.
I couldn't quite fathom what I was seeing until I was greeted with
the poster of H, who I had gone to school with: she had been my
partner in food tech throughout Year 9. I hadn't seen her in years.
Starting to cry, I raced on ahead, desperate to reach the office.

When I arrived, I found out that overnight it had been transformed into a donation hub. Normal work had come to a halt;
there were no desks to sit at, and I put an out-of-office reply
on my email, saying something vague about not being available
due to 'unforeseen circumstances'. At the time we thought it
was a small fire, and that we could support the victims by
bringing together random bits and bobs. One of my tasks
involved organising all of those donations. It took a while for
us to realise the extent of the fire; that a lot of the people on
the posters hadn't managed to escape the burning tower. They
weren't in hospitals across London – they hadn't made it out.
Eventually we had a church full of clothes with no one to give
them to because there simply weren't enough survivors for
them to be useful. It was a sombre realisation that would stay
with me for the months that followed.

While there were things we didn't know in that initial phase,
it became clear very soon that this event would highlight some
of the best, and the worst things about my city, and this country.
The fire very quickly became a massive news spectacle, with
politicians and press descending on the grieving community.
My job then grew to include guarding the doors of the rooms
where bereaved families grieved or dealt with the gruelling
bureaucracy that comes with tragedy. Once, a family who had
lost their infant son sat behind one of those doors, and in my
job letting in family members to support them I had to turn
away a journalist who had hidden his camera, pretending to be
kin. I managed to contain the almost overwhelming urge to
yell at him, and I'll never forget how he walked away so
unashamedly. On another day, a Kensington mother – the *other*
Kensington – arrived with her daughter. It was half-term, and
she thought she would 'bring her along to help out and learn
about community values'. I watched as they managed to fix

two donation packages, then took their phones out and began taking photos of themselves, posting on social media about their 'work'. Unfortunately, this type of volunteer was relatively common, but I said nothing: I had no energy left for those types of people.

My role evolved as the needs of the survivors became clearer. The charity I worked at, along with many other voluntary groups, decided to provide the support the government was unwilling to give. Overnight I became a caseworker, sitting with people who had escaped the tower and helping them fill out grotesquely elaborate forms in order to claim £250 or £500 for themselves and their families. The process was cruel: one of the questions asked them to detail what they had lost in the fire, and so they would sit, fresh from the trauma of the blaze, and attempt to list in black ink the heirlooms, mementos, furniture, machines and clothes that had been blackened to ash and smoke. I felt responsible for their tears in that moment. Still, there were others who would hug me afterwards, immensely grateful for my help, which didn't feel right either. While I was appreciative of their thanks, these people had been failed – by the state, and by society – and their total gratitude at a small kindness made me uneasy.

Regardless, the people liked and trusted me. We would make small talk; I'd ask them where they were from, and then they would ask me. With their trust came vulnerability on both sides – it was the first time I started talking to people openly about my own identity, too. They started calling for 'the Afghan girl' to help them out – a small comfort for them, I imagine, when faced with my mostly white colleagues. The comfort people felt around me created a space where they could be honest about their pain. I remember Billy – a pensioner who had lived near Grenfell for decades – talking to me outside one day and telling me that despite the sweltering summer heat, he couldn't bear to keep his window open any more.

'I just hear screams,' he said. 'That night, I heard so many screams, and now if I hear the tiniest voice outside my window, I jump up thinking it's people screaming. I can't stop berating myself about how I could have done more – should have done more.'

The experiences of the survivors were unimaginable, and so I began to hold their trust, grief and vulnerability in my twenty-two-year-old body. It was unbearably heavy, but every day I would force myself to keep it together and carry it with me on the bus, until I got home. Only then would the bundle unravel, and I would spend hours crying, because it was just so much. The trauma of Grenfell was ever-present – television, social media, text messages from friends – and inescapable, even when sobbing alone in my room. I lived with my family at the time, but I didn't share much about what was happening as I didn't want them to worry about me or feel what I was being made to feel. I avoided telling people that the smoking tombstone was essentially now my workplace: it would have felt as if I was leaking the stories the survivors had trusted me with. Personal accounts were being so twisted by the media, with some far-right groups saying they had deserved it. The sadness and isolation I felt started to grow, penetrating deeper and lasting longer, becoming more than just a reaction to the work I was doing. My eventual depression looked in some ways like the typical picture: me, alone, in a dark room with the curtains closed. At my lowest moments, I would lose all motivation and any sense of hope. And quite quickly I would start catastrophising – believing only the worst outcomes were possible in any given situation. I felt truly and utterly deactivated, like I just couldn't make things work.

Something about this event and this work was affecting me deeply, more than it affected my white colleagues. Working with these survivors – Black and Brown people, people who spoke many languages; people who had left homes behind in other countries, only to lose it again here; these people who faced ambivalence at best, and hostility at worst from a state that was complicit in their trauma – started to scrape at the story buried inside me, which until then I had left untouched and unexamined. It became harder and harder for me to cope, until I felt myself spiralling into despair as the pain of their stories got tangled up with my own.

My family arrived in the UK from Kabul in 2000. I don't remember Afghanistan too much, but I picture the landscape the way my parents describe it: the Himalayas on the horizon, the clear rivers, the way the seasons change so completely, bringing sandy heat, lush green, and icy white with a conviction we lack in England. In my mind, it's powerful, beautiful and vast, all the way down to the fruit – to this day my dad still talks about the impressively large watermelons and oranges.

Afghan Sikhs have lived in Afghanistan for centuries and my parents got married in Gurdwara Karte Parwan in Kabul. Their wedding video follows them from the ceremony to my grandparents' house, where they celebrated surrounded by Hindu, Muslim and Sikh friends and family. My favourite part is in between, as they are driven in a flower-laden car with the Hindu Kush mountains behind them, and the sound of the Bollywood song 'Kabhi Bhoola Kabhi Yaad Kiya' in the background. As of summer 2022, Gurdwara Karte Parwan has been blasted to rubble after years of bombing, its remnants now abandoned.

My dad was a merchant, of sorts. A proud Sikh man with a turban, he would travel to Russia to sell clothes and other household items in markets across the border. He still speaks Russian fluently. Mum was a housewife – a typical life for a young Afghan Sikh woman. She mostly stayed in the confines of home, well aware that venturing into the streets unchaperoned was unwise.

Things changed when the Mujahedeen, and later Taliban, came into power. Sikhs were made to wear a yellow band in public and Gurdwaras started getting attacked. Without spaces for Sikhs to gather, worship and live safely, the community was in existential danger. Figures are hard to come by, but from likely hundreds of thousands of Sikh families in Afghanistan pre-1992, fewer than a couple of hundred now remain.

My parents decided to leave with me and my older sister when I was five. I don't remember much about the decision; I just remember having to pack stuff. I don't think any of us were prepared for the long and traumatic journey: we were simply told to pay the smugglers, and that they would get us across. We filled two or three bags of essentials: a light load, leaving the rest of our belongings behind. My mum – like many Afghan Sikhs – kept her money in gold, and carefully packed away the earrings that would be part of our seed on arrival somewhere safe and new. I remember the first meeting with the people-smugglers on the route. We had to travel light and I remember so clearly them picking up our suitcases and just tossing them away, right over their heads. Twenty-two years later, my mum still remembers that moment – that feeling of losing everything you have in an instant, and just having to keep on moving to save whatever you have left. It's a feeling that I saw again and again during Grenfell in the hands of parents picking up food parcels, or signing names on forms, and heard in their voices as they asked what they should do until their financial support came through from the government.

'I ran away from a war to come to this country, and this feels worse than a war. My house is up in flames,' a woman said to me in Kensington. It seems obvious, now, that offering to support the survivors of the Grenfell fire would affect me in the way that it did, but I was unable to link the two until I went to therapy.

My mental health was rapidly deteriorating: I'd begun to withdraw, I was no longer replying to friends messaging me, I stopped eating regular meals. My only relief was on my journey home from work, where I would allow myself to cry the tears I'd bottled up all day. Fortunately, I was able to access support through some donations to my workplace. It was in those sessions that I began to explore why working in the aftermath of Grenfell had been so triggering for me, to the point that I handed in my notice within a few months of the fire. I continued to interrogate this with a different therapist after I left that role, using a therapeutic technique called 'narrative exposure therapy'. Over a year and a half, we mapped out my entire life, from birth to the present day, and spent sessions working through all of the major traumatic events. It was hard going, but vital.

I realised there was a lot about my own story that I had either forgotten or buried, consciously or unconsciously. Memories came back to me: being held at gunpoint by smugglers looking for the dregs of cash we had left; running through forests and hiding on the sides of roads. Memories of being in a lorry, all of us ill after weeks of travelling and sleeping outside, with my mum holding her clothes over my mouth so the driver wouldn't hear me cough, and of arriving in Dover and jumping out, wearing all four of the outfits that I owned, each layered haphazardly on top of the other.

Some of these memories felt new, but there were others I'd always remembered. From the moment of our arrival, life in the

UK was not straightforward. We arrived in the year 2000; the following year, the 9/11 attacks sparked the War on Terror. As asylum seekers we were initially settled in Newcastle, and we experienced racist attacks. One of my first memories is being pulled by the hair off a swing in the local park by two girls – bearing in mind how important hair is to Sikhs. They called me 'a Taliban', and told me to get out of *their* country. My dad, still proudly wearing his turban, would regularly get similar abuse. Eventually we moved to London, where we lived with family for a while, until we were housed in our own place. Some struggles remained, though – my dad spent years repaying the money he had borrowed to get us out of Afghanistan, and my mum struggled to learn English, with ESOL classes having their funding slashed – a problem migrants still face today.

School was difficult – the white kids didn't want to be my friend – but home was also sad, with Mum going through her own depression and Dad struggling to find work. Within all of that, though, there was also some joy: Ahmad Zahir – the 'Elvis of Afghanistan' – playing in the background; my parents telling stories about my grandparents to my two younger siblings who were born here, and never got to meet them. An enduring source of joy from that time came from learning English, and then learning to read – books became my friends. I'd go home with stacks of them, racing through new worlds and falling in love with new characters. In my teenage years I discovered books by Afghan authors, and in a way I got to relive part of my past through them, sharing the street names from *The Kite Runner* with my dad and hearing his memories of them as a teenager himself.

As I grew, my mind did what it needed to protect me: certain memories were left behind in favour of others. Grenfell changed that, and in the immediate aftermath, I was retraumatised by flashbacks of my past with no real way of processing them. Therapy allowed me to open up Pandora's box – to rediscover my history, and understand how the different parts joined up together to form an elaborate patchwork. It's helped me understand the way I am: I know where I come from, what I've been through, what I have to live with, why certain things can trigger me so easily; in short I have a better understanding of what makes me, me.

Still, moving through the world with a fuller knowledge of what has happened to me is hard, though thankfully I now have the tools to make adjustments to my life to better help me live with my complex PTSD. I currently work in the equalities sector, which can be heavy, and a small win has been to successfully request to work from home, since my good and bad days can be so unpredictable without the added pressure of heading into an office every day. Understanding myself better has also helped my relationships. I used to avoid talking about Afghanistan, and my childhood, for fear of bringing down the mood of the people around me. I've now learned that if I can be relaxed about it, others will usually follow my lead. I met my partner three years ago, and it was the first time I'd told a partner about my history – he's white, middle class, and in many ways his life experience couldn't be more different – and yet, with him, it was empowering not to distance myself from my story. I can see now how it has formed so much of my identity: the empathy I feel for certain people and the passion I have for my work were shaped by my lived experience.

When I look in the mirror, I see the five-year-old who stumbled out of the back of a lorry. I feel like she's watching me, and I owe it to her to do well with what I have now. I used to shy away from conversations about my background because I didn't understand it. It felt like a messy, dark hole, but through therapy I can visualise it. I can see that five-year-old, clear as day. It's like I've arranged the chaotic jumble of papers floating in my head and slotted them into neat files. I can pull a memory when I need to, talk about it, then slot it back in. Coming to terms with trauma is hard, and I still get depressed many days of the week, but I feel much more whole. I understand myself in a way I never thought I would.

Therapy worked well for me, but finding the right type of therapy, and the right therapist took time. Naturally, the power and social dynamics of the therapeutic encounter reflect those of the outside world, and for me, this sometimes meant uncomfortable or simply offensive interactions in a space where I was supposed to be healing from racism, rather than encountering it. In the aftermath of Grenfell the therapy I received was funded by my workplace and included group sessions with my majority white colleagues. They had all helped in the relief effort, and in doing so had experienced their own trauma, but navigating the legitimate issues we were experiencing was complicated by the threads of white saviourism that entered the sessions.

For similar reasons, the racial identity of the therapist themselves has affected my ability to participate effectively in it. I've changed therapists four or five times, largely because they made insensitive comments, and I struggled to eventually find a therapist of colour who could deal with my issues with the care and sensitivity they required. The comments ranged from the alienating ('Oh, I've never met someone from Afghanistan, how fascinating!') to the victim-blaming ('Your mum has lived here for twenty-two years and hasn't bothered learning the language? Doesn't that make you angry?').

There were things that a person of colour would take as a given whereas a white therapist would need explaining or even convincing. Like the fact that for some people – poor, Brown, women, refugees – the outside world can be a dangerous place, whether that's because you've been persecuted as a religious minority in Afghanistan, bundled in secret across Europe, or racially abused in the streets of England as a new arrival. Having to explain and justify my mum's trauma, rather than challenge the social and political factors that led to her situation was an offensive distraction from the healing progress I was trying to engage in. Finding a therapist of colour meant that there was a level of understanding that allowed me to talk without explanation, caveats or disclaimers. I was able to relax enough to unpick issues I hadn't been able to until that point, because I hadn't felt safe to do so.

I've been fortunate enough to be able to access private therapists, but this isn't the case for many people who need long-term psychological support. Unfortunately, psychological therapy in the NHS is under-funded and under-resourced, and as for so many others, my attempts to access therapy on the NHS have been met with long waiting lists, with the only option at the end of the tunnel being a short course in cognitive behavioural therapy. CBT is a really useful therapy for lots of people, but I found it frustrating to try to explain to my GP how my complex trauma would not be served by it. At times it felt like they failed to understand what I required, and other friends have had similar issues. In many cases, the lack of funding forces a one-size-fits-all approach, which is the opposite of the tailored, long-term support needed to get to the root of the mental health issues caused by complex and enduring trauma. I'm glad I got the therapy I needed, but I despair for others like me – and perhaps Grenfell survivors included – who have been unable to get the affordable, sensitive, tailored therapy that they also need.

*

The terror has always been inside me: of being five years old, the youngest of a family of refugees, traversing Europe with only the clothes on our backs. With Grenfell, I was confronted by the cruelty of the life – and death – that too often awaits families like mine once they arrive in a place they hope to call home. In retrospect it was inevitable that such a catastrophic event would bring to the surface my own long-suppressed trauma, and force me to begin learning to console that terrified five-year-old. This was difficult, and the period immediately after the Grenfell fire was dark for me, but I'm also proud of what I achieved in helping the survivors, and later on myself, to move forward. Hard times continue, and unexpected challenges seem to always be around the corner. For example, I'm on antidepressants now, and they give me the most intense, vivid dreams. I can spend a night being chased and beheaded by the Taliban and wake up unable to begin my day in the real world, and I just have to stay in bed until I can manage. Certain triggers will throw me off balance, and I'll be dragged back to bad times from my childhood. Things can feel pointless, and when I'm catastrophising I can feel suicidal. I'm still not able to talk to my family about my mental health or my therapy, because of the stigma they still associate with it, and I also don't want to upset them with how much I've struggled. Even finding the language for a conversation about mental health with my parents would be difficult, as we aren't used to discussing it at home. Beyond that, the idea of talking about my problems with a therapist is alien and would be discouraged: airing our dirty laundry to outsiders is something my family has always steered away from. Regardless, food is the way my mum shows me love, and when I am feeling down (and unable to cook), I can always rely on her Tupperware tubs full of delicious curries for some comfort.

I'm still learning about myself, and my mental health. Right now, my depression is manifesting in the form of feeling unhinged and ungrounded. I think it's a feeling a lot of immigrants experience – a duality of having to get on with life in the UK, and putting the other side of you on hold; the side where difficult things might have happened which are related to your other identity. I think Grenfell was so triggering for me because this tragedy in a tower block in Kensington somehow mirrored my past, and forced me to face that other identity. It made me reflect on my place in the world as a young woman of colour, and a refugee. The pain was familiar, but it wasn't something that was supposed to happen here. When people ask me where I'm from and I say Afghanistan, the replies are often strange. 'Jokes' about how I must not have been back home for a holiday in a while, or allusions to the rhetoric of the news and films that it's a horrible, unliveable war zone; a place of danger, unlike the UK. The undeniable violence of Grenfell in a leafy borough of west London caused me to reflect on my past in Afghanistan. The tragedy should serve to remind us that suffering, violence and neglect happen routinely, insidiously, and on a societal level right in front of us in the UK. The policies that leave people starving during a cost of living crisis, or children unable to access mental health services, or my mum too scared to feel safe on her own out in London are all of our problem, and require a reckoning of the inequalities and power dynamics at play in our society. I used to tell my therapist how ridiculous it was that it took a building burning down for me to sit down and talk about my own trauma; for the sake of everyone in tower blocks across the country, I hope it only takes one for our society to do the same.

# Ready to Fly

## Cat

### As told to Shelley Harris

This is not a sob story. I want you to understand what it's like for me to be a doctor with a mental illness. I want you to understand what it's like for me to be human. I have promised myself that I will speak the truth with my whole heart, so I'm going to tell you everything.

I'm going to tell you about the moment when, as a junior doctor, I presented myself at the hospital's front desk and said: I work here, and I want to kill myself.

But before I do, there are some other things I want you to know about me. Growing up, I was the class entertainer. I had an intense desire to make things better for people, to fix what was broken, and at that age my preferred way of achieving it was by providing distraction. Later, as a medical trainee, there were other ways to help; I was at a festival once and spotted, silhouetted on a hillside, the unmistakeable movements of someone trying to administer CPR. I rushed up the slope and did everything I could to save the patient. I did not succeed.

That's another thing you should know: failure doesn't scare me, and because of this I've had brilliant adventures. I've gone on an expedition to a wild and isolated place; I've written award-winning poetry; I've narrowly missed being caught in an avalanche in the foothills of Nepal; I've stood alone onstage and shared my lived experience with an audience of strangers. The value that means the most to me is courage.

I want you to know all these things because another thing about me is that I have a mental illness. It matters very much to me that I'm not seen wholly through that lens.

I work as a psychiatrist now, for lots of excellent reasons. There's my desire to help, which has never gone away. There's also the fact that I treasure human stories. That's what you're trusted with as a psychiatrist; every single one of them is a gift. And if all human stories are important, mine is too.

This is my story.

There's no clear place where it begins, so I'm going to begin when I applied to medical school. I look back now to teenage me and I'm honestly a bit baffled about my motivation. Why medicine? I wanted to make the world better and, urged on by my pushy grammar school, thought that this would be a good way to do it. At my interview I remember telling the dean of the medical school, 'I'm doing this because I want to help.' I didn't know what my statement really meant, or what I might be capable of. What do we know, at seventeen?

On the first day of university I changed my name – from Catherine to Cat – because my closest school friends called me Cat and I thought: if everyone here calls me that, everyone will be my friend. It was an incredibly stimulating environment. I worked flat out and did well. And though not all my fellow students fell for the Cat strategy, enough of them did that I made lifelong friendships.

Looking back, I can see that the problems I experienced in

my third year were red flags. After two years of academic study, clinical training had started. I was sent to a hospital to meet real patients with real needs – and in real distress and pain. I'd said I wanted to help people, and now here they were, waiting for me to help them.

I began suffering from anxiety, and sometimes more than anxiety. Sometimes, I found myself in the grip of an over-whelming flood of terror. I'd be assailed by a conviction of impending doom – right here, right now – and knew I had to escape. *I'm going to shout*, I'd think. *I'm about to scream and go crazy and make a fool of myself. Get out!* If I was in a lecture I'd 'sorry' my way along the row of desks and run out of the room, dash for the loos and sit on the floor of a cubicle, paralysed until my friends came to find me.

I'd feel all those things on the wards of the hospital, too, watching experienced doctors at work. It often happened when I was about to help out with an intricate, difficult procedure, especially if it might cause suffering. But I never left the room – not once. Just stayed put, feeling all the feelings, keeping them locked inside.

I now know how to name these events: I was having panic attacks. At the time, even as a medical student, there was a sort of mental barrier; I just couldn't identify what was happening. Instead I saw a doctor, got a prescription for beta blockers – which manage superficial, physical symptoms – and on I went.

At the end of my fifth year I experienced a catastrophic failure, the sort of failure you think will send you into freefall if your mental health is already shaky. We'd taken our final written tests and I'd done well. The last barrier to becoming a doctor was the practical exam. I was determined to pass with flying colours. I got together with a group of friends and we worked all hours to revise, sometimes in ingenious ways. I remember filling a sandwich bag with hot chocolate, tucking it under my jumper so that when my partner did an abdominal exam they'd find the 'colostomy bag' on me; we constructed homemade testicles for the genitalia exam; we rigged a timer with a buzzing klaxon to a huge pair of speakers, so it would blast out when time was up for each question. When results day came I stood amongst my friends, everyone ripping open their results letters. I ripped open mine.

I'd failed.

I was devastated. I remember bursting into tears and torturing myself by reading everyone's celebratory Facebook posts. But what surprised me is that it . . . was OK. Failure didn't kill me. It didn't even scar me. I gathered myself, did the retake, passed. I started work as a junior doctor. That's why I don't fear failure: because I *did* fail – badly, at a critical point in my life – and I'm still standing.

Things were good after that, even when shift patterns were atrocious, even when I was painfully aware of my own limitations. I worked, I learned, I gained experience. As I became more capable, my self-esteem increased; there's something hugely sustaining about becoming competent. I was scared of the job and I loved it, all at once.

Then I got an amazing opportunity – to travel on an expedition as the team medic. We'd be in a remote location and would have to fend for ourselves, eating only what we caught or grew, living under shelter we'd constructed. We'd be pushed to our physical limits and far from everything we'd known, but it was a once-in-a-lifetime chance. I grabbed it with both hands.

At first, things went well. I threw myself into the expedition, and into my role of growing food for the team. I was homesick, but that wasn't out of the ordinary – everyone was homesick. Then, two months in, among strangers and far from medical help (correction: I *was* the medical help), things began to go wrong.

It happened slowly at first: things just a little out of kilter. Not so much that you'd worry. Not so much that you'd understand what was happening. It began with sleep. I'd wake, energised, at 4 a.m., despite having exhausted myself the previous day. I was dreaming vividly, dreams rich with emotion, which bled into the next morning; I remember one in which I missed my family with a deep, desperate grief and woke in the small hours, face wet with tears. As soon as I got up, I'd write in my journal. I still have that notebook, pages crammed with lines and lines of tiny, tiny, tiny handwriting: top to bottom, edge to edge, jammed tight with the insights I'd gained. Or I'd make a video, gabbling nonstop to record all the wisdom I needed to share – I couldn't talk fast enough. Then I'd go and watch the sunrise.

I remember one morning in particular, sitting cross-legged on a sand dune, watching the sun come up. As it rose, I became filled – every part of me completely suffused – with a transcendent knowledge. With enlightenment. I wept, knowing that everything was going to be OK. My life would be utterly changed now, because I was like the Buddha, exactly like him, and I didn't need to eat any more, or depend on anyone or anything, ever again. I could just sit there forever and *be*.

That's the thing about mania. It gives you all the epiphanies.

My transcendence lasted until the other expedition members woke. Wrenched back into the world, I was shocked out of my state, and it was then that my medical education kicked in: this was not normal. I even tentatively identified what I was experiencing. Seeking confirmation, I went to my room and opened my notebook. When I saw the words filling the most recent pages, it seemed to me that I hadn't written them at all.

All of this, I kept from the others. But things were getting harder. I started to feel threatened, then paranoid. We set out in a boat to catch fish, and I suddenly found that I didn't really know the people I was with. They were strangers, dangerous predators, and we were getting further from the shore. It would be easy for them to throw me from the boat and drown me. Yes – that was it. That was what they were going to do.

These thoughts, and others like them, came relentlessly. I had to leave, but telling the truth seemed impossible. Instead, I formulated plans that seem outlandish now, but at the time made sense. I would break my leg, I decided. (I would scrabble across high rocks, and pretend to lose my balance, and fall and crack my bones.) Then they'd have to evacuate me for reasons of physical injury. Better that than being the 'madwoman' of the expedition.

In a calmer moment, I found the courage to tell the truth – part of it, anyway. In the midst of the delusions and paranoia, I'm proud that I managed to be at least that honest. I told them I had to leave, and then I left.

I went back to where I'd grown up. My parents had been travelling, but some instinct had told them to come back to Britain. In my delusions I'd imagined them as dead. No, as not quite dead. Still alive, but totally disconnected from me. The conviction had taken hold, to the point that it didn't even disturb me any more; it was established fact. I'd accepted it peacefully, continuing life without them. And now here they were, meeting me off the train! I was ecstatic. Mum and Dad were reincarnated, brand new to me as I would be to them: fresh from the expedition – dishevelled, a mess, a wild feral woman. We would get to know each other all over again.

I went home, but I almost wish I hadn't, because of what came next.

There were some good times in those first few days; I'd listen to records with my dad, reconnecting with him. I decided, in one of my epiphanies, that I was ready to become a mother. But other thoughts were more troubling. My grandmother had died, and when Dad took me to the bank to confirm my inheritance, I didn't trust him to counter-sign the document. Those notebooks I'd filled during the expedition? I carried them everywhere. At night, I refused to sleep in my bed, having not slept in one for four months by that point. In fact, I didn't sleep at all for the first few days; it was like my eyes were wide awake. I didn't nod or doze, just watched the movement of the clock's second hand, which had itself started to behave oddly, sometimes ticking as normal, sometimes racing round its circle, over and over again: a minute passing in a few seconds, an hour in moments.

One day, my mum and I went to look at the house she and my dad had bought while I was away, and I became convinced that I was in a lucid dream, where you move through the experience fully conscious of your dreaming state. I was being led somewhere important. When the door opened, my whole family – all the dead, all the living – would be waiting behind it to greet me. When that didn't happen, when Mum instead led me away, the door unopened, it was devastating. We got home and my distress ramped up. I asked to see a doctor. Mum tried to comfort me with a cup of tea but I didn't touch it, certain that she and Dad were imposters, that she'd laced it with poison, these thoughts assailing me even as I heard her on the phone to the GP, begging for an appointment. When they said it wasn't possible I got more desperate, demanding to go to A & E.

We drove there through a landscape alive with meaning: traffic lights and road names carrying coded significance, road signs sending messages, songs on the car radio talking to me.

When we arrived, the TV in the waiting room was on, broadcasting secret communications – for my eyes only.

Thank God, I thought, when we finally saw a doctor, when that doctor recognised that I was having a psychotic episode. Thank God. I can't do this all by myself.

But they didn't have any beds, so they sent me home with a prescription for diazepam, a drug that calms you in times of crisis. At the pharmacy, I was lost in delusions (I wasn't a doctor after all, but a fake. In medical school, I'd murdered my flatmates). Back at home, I thought I was still in a dream and that, to get out of it, I had to overdose on the diazepam: I had to die in the nightmare, so I could wake into the real world. Mum had the pills so I went for her, trying to grab them. We fought, fierce and awkward, each completely determined – I to get the tablets, she to stop me. When she wouldn't let go, I filched my wallet and passport, slipped them into my pocket and did a runner, bellowing for help. Dad hauled me into the house, kicking and screaming. Back we went then, to the same hospital but a different department – the mental health centre. This time we refused to leave until I got help.

Which was how I finally did get help.

I stayed as an inpatient, took the diazepam, slept, and sleep itself was a curative of sorts, my mind bent out of shape by so many days without it. I woke in a better state, and after that took a few months off to recover. 'Recovery' in this case meant medication – not the medication I really needed, as it turned out, but an antidepressant which allowed me to return to something approaching normal. I completed my second year as a junior doctor, back where I'd worked before. But I still hadn't been diagnosed and my thoughts were chaotic. I cooked up a sketchy plan to turn my back on medicine completely and train as a yoga teacher instead. I'd do that in India, I decided.

I set a date to put my things into storage and leave the country. When the day came, I found myself overwhelmed by emotions and false memories. Some might call this delusional; I would call it a psychotic reaction triggered by acute stress, much as I'd had when I'd left the expedition. Unable to cope with all these feelings, I began to experience suicidal urges.

My car crammed with possessions, I took a detour to the hospital where I worked. It had a lake. I was going to drown myself in it. After parking, I looked across the grounds to where the lake waited. I looked at the hospital entrance. And in a last attempt to save my own life, I went towards those doors.

This, you may remember, is where we began. I went up to the receptionist and said: 'I work here, and I want to kill myself.' Because here's the truth of it: when you're suicidal, you don't want to die. You just need the unbearable feelings to stop.

Before things got better, they got worse. I was kept in overnight. My parents were called. I spent the time screaming in distress, and my parents . . . my parents had to see and hear all of it.

I find it hard to get past that memory. It overwhelms me, even now.

When that dreadful night was over, I was sectioned and got a diagnosis of bipolar affective disorder. At the time, I accepted the diagnosis. I recognised that I now carried a new label, and felt it was for the best. The diagnosis allowed me access to new drugs – I was prescribed a mood stabiliser – and to begin ten days of inpatient treatment. From there, recovery was . . . the way recovery usually is: a trend upwards, but only when you stand back and look from afar (from the future, maybe, like I am now). Close to, it's up and down, steps forward and back.

After hospital came three weeks at a halfway house, which

offered supported independence. Then I made some decisions about my future.

I moved to a new city; Dad helped me find a house there. I applied for a part-time master's degree in public health and was accepted, so then I had some direction. To pay my way, I got on the books of a locum agency. Locums are doctors who fill in as substitutes when there's a staff shortage; in my case, I got ad hoc shifts in elderly care. By now I'd been out of hospital for two months. And in between study and the job and finding my way, I began to write.

I was in my car one day, when words suddenly came to me in the form of a rhyme. I had written songs before, but I'm not much of a singer, so I'd never had a place to put them. I knew this was going to be a poem.

When I write poetry, the flow of words comes naturally into my brain. Sometimes I have to write it down immediately. At other times I filter it and form the rhythm until it's a finished piece. The words can always be edited, so there is no harm in writing them down and seeing what happens.

The next part needed a lot of courage. I went to an open mic night (my first – I had no idea how these things worked) and read my poem to the audience. Utter terror, but . . . they liked it. In fact, talking openly about mental health even seemed to strike a chord. So I performed in other places, growing in confidence all the time, and the poem ended up winning an award at a mental health arts festival. This was my first taste of performance poetry, and I was immediately addicted.

When the locum position started to feel overwhelming, I stepped away from it and got a job with a local charity, supporting sex workers. My clients had lots of mental health issues and I felt like I could relate. I found that when they opened up about how they were feeling, I was able to put myself in their shoes. I began to see how my own experiences could support other people.

At the same time I was having therapy, finishing the master's, making friends; I was rebuilding my life. It was a slow process, as these things are. I was also continuing to write. I became a regular at open mic nights, splurging my words to the audiences, eventually becoming a finalist in a national competition and performing at the Royal Albert Hall. I loved having a platform to speak about my experiences and tell my story to a room of people listening intently. It felt good. It felt like a brave thing to do.

After the charity role I got a job in an office, which was a turning point for me. Not because I loved it – quite the opposite. I was unimaginably bored, and that boredom propelled me into practising medicine again; I wanted to apply my hard-won skills. By now it was about three years since my hospital stay. I knew what it felt like to help other people with mental illness, coming from a place of empathy and lived experience, and I applied for training as a psychiatrist, not really believing I'd get the job. But I did – the joy! – and that's what I'm doing now: working part-time as a psychiatrist, leaving myself space to manage my condition and develop my writing. In the midst of all that, there's been a twist I didn't see coming.

I started sessions of cognitive analytical therapy, and not long after that began working on the story you're reading right now. To my therapist I talked about my life as it currently is, but I've also spent weeks talking and writing about my past experiences, recounting them to the author I've teamed up with for this project. In the process, something has shifted. I've realised that my symptoms may not after all fit the 'bipolar' label. Finally, as this book was going to press, I mentioned those reservations to my therapist, who agreed and suggested that, instead of bipolar disorder, I may be suffering from post-traumatic stress disorder

(PTSD), brought on by my experiences during the expedition.

When we get a diagnosis it's tempting to see it as something written in stone, but my experience as a doctor shows me that changes in diagnosis are far from unusual. I haven't yet received a formal confirmation of PTSD, but if I do it may mean that I don't need to take medication at all. Instead, I'll receive specialist trauma-based therapy to help me process events, and my therapist will help me manage my symptoms without antipsychotics.

All of this is very new to me, but it also feels right. I'm experiencing a huge mixture of emotions. There's anxiety about the diagnosis change, because I'd partially accepted that I had bipolar – though taking the medication always felt wrong somehow. I also feel anger at having been stuck with a label, and the wrong one at that. But I also feel . . . hopeful. Like I'm on the right path.

This isn't just about me as a patient, though; it feeds into my practice as a doctor. For want of a better word, it's made me more 'enlightened' as a psychiatrist. In the future, I'll think – and investigate – more carefully than ever, before placing labels on my patients.

I was hesitant at first about taking part in this book, about 'coming out' as a doctor with a mental illness. In the past, some have suffered for doing that. One GP, who was open about having bipolar, received abuse from her patients and ended up killing herself. She must have felt so trapped and exposed, and I bet she wished she'd never spoken out. But if a doctor had cancer or a broken leg, they wouldn't agonise about disclosing it – why should having a mental disorder be any different? I have done everything I can to help myself with this condition – a condition I did not ask for and that isn't my fault. I shouldn't have to be silent about it.

In fact, I think my experiences with mental illness have made me a far *better* medic than the one I was before; my knowledge base is much broader than that of your average junior doctor. I don't tell patients that I have a mental disorder and currently take the same medication they do, because the last thing I want is to diminish their experiences by talking about my own. But when manic patients have epiphanies – I've been there. When depressed patients are suicidal – I've been there. I get it. Approaching patients with empathy is very different from the attitude I took when I was a medical student. Then, I found some of these presentations bizarre, but now I understand them from the inside. In a way, this makes me grateful to have been through the pain.

There's one final benefit of being a psychiatrist with a mental illness. After everything I've been through, I have hope for my patients. Hope is a precious and vital thing. It can be hard to find when you're in the midst of a mental health crisis. I've felt what it's like when things are at their worst, when you can't imagine them improving . . . and then I've seen them improve. Things can get better. I know they can, because they did for me.

My responsibility goes beyond the way I interact with patients; I also advocate for mental health amongst fellow doctors. One of the bravest moments of my life was when I called out another junior doctor who was about to work on the psychiatric wards and referred to the patients as 'crazies'. Another time, a surgeon told me that psychiatry shouldn't be part of the medical field. I think back to these colleagues, wondering about the experiences their own patients have had with co-morbid physical health issues and mental illness (because they *will* have had them). That junior doctor wanted to work in intensive care. Some of his patients will wake up in ITU having attempted to take their own lives, and his will be the first face they see.

As for those other doctors who suffer from mental illness, I hope my openness helps them, too. I know four who have died by suicide. There's a real danger in constructing an identity that is solely about caring for others, because it becomes impossible to ask for help. Doctors are at the top of the caring ladder, and sometimes we think the only way down is to jump. Instead, we should go down one rung at a time and allow people to support us as we do them.

Beyond work, my life is busy and sociable, full of novelty. Anxiety can be paralysing when you're thinking of taking up something new, but my secret weapon is that I've already had to face my two biggest fears. In the past, my worst anxieties centred on not being good enough, and on the possibility of 'going crazy'. But after everything I've experienced, I've realised that I *am* good enough. As for 'going crazy' – well, I did that. So now, when the things I want to achieve are beyond my reach, I have a go anyway.

On top of all this, managing my condition is a full-time job. There's ordering medication and remembering to take it, a daily reminder of the unpleasant fact that to continue living in this world I need to take pills for my brain (until the doctors tell me I can stop). I work hard to manage my emotions and regulate my mood.

To help do this, I've built a support network. It's more fun than it sounds, because I've filled up my life with people who inspire and sustain me – and I'm as open as possible with them about my feelings. Most days I will check in, usually starting with a 'how's things?' message as a way of kick-starting the conversation.

As I learn new things about myself, I revise and edit my Wellness Recovery Action Plan, an A4 card containing a list of my routine daily tasks, my triggers, my crisis plan and post-crisis plan. Finally, I need to keep appointments with the psychiatrists, counsellors, community nurses and GP who professionally support me.

It is gruelling having a mental illness but if I didn't do these things I wouldn't be able to cope. In the past, when my life has gone out of balance, I've ended up being admitted to psychiatric hospital, a place I only want to enter as a doctor who can make things better for others.

Having a mental illness is not a tragedy. It is neither a blessing nor a curse, but a unique state of mind – one that has, for me, brought great creativity. And when I do feel low in mood, what I need from my support network is help with practicalities. Making sure I'm cared for, prompting me to do basic things like washing, eating and getting what I need into the house.

As I come out of a low period, I usually find something to take hold of: a new interest that can be harnessed and used as energy to continue. Past interests include volunteering at a forest school with young kids, sea swimming and an obsession with the vagus nerve – the part of the nervous system that helps us to relax.

In psychiatry, we talk about the 'premorbid personality' – what a patient was like before their mental illness episode. When you come out of that episode, you have undergone a change, but the former 'you' is still there. It's hard – but incredibly helpful – to hold on to that when the clouds descend. It turns out that I like the person I am now, as well as the one I used to be. I fully anticipate liking future me, too.

Who knows what will come next? I continue to work as a part-time psychiatrist and I write every day and perform poetry. I'm so glad that I dared to explore the artistic side of myself. I'm happy that I have had the courage to speak out about what happened to me, and about the ways in which all of us – as individuals and communities – can tackle poor mental health.

That's what led me to do this project, and to share my lived experience with you.

I wonder at times where I would be if none of this had happened. But you play the cards you are dealt, and though being human is hard, even difficult events bring with them advantages. I'm thankful that I have food in the fridge and shelter above my head. I'm even grateful for oxygen. During those times when I'm stuck in bed, paralysed with low mood, I work my way up from those most basic of needs to higher ones: I have breath in my lungs, I have food in my body, I have rest and sleep, and eventually I will emerge from my cocoon – transformed, and ready to fly.

# Elements of a Breakdown

## Phoenix

### As told to Hafsa Zayyan

She remembers the feeling of Rosy on her back. Small, soft and warm. Rosy is giggling uncontrollably as she spins round and round in circles in the long grass. The sun is creating black spots behind her eyes. Dandelion seeds are flying everywhere; into their mouths, up their noses. She starts to sneeze and loses her balance and the pair of them, lumped together like a hunchback, fall to the ground. She panics, but Rosy is not hurt. She's clambering on top of her, tugging at the lapels of her stupid school shirt, saying: again, again, again! She thinks she holds so much power in this moment, but even then, it's really Rosy who wields the power. This is the moment she wants to remember. This is the best moment of her life.

She worries that she is dying. A tiny voice inside her tells her this: her instinct. The pain comes and goes in waves; sometimes it is tolerable; mostly, it is not. Imagine your insides are a cotton cloth held between two people and twisted in opposite directions until that cloth becomes a small, hard ball. That is what it feels like is happening to her stomach.

171

Hospitals smell like bleach and decay and food from the school canteen that has been sitting out for too long. She hates this smell the way she hates people biting their fingernails. It makes her feel physically sick. So every time she has to go to hospital, she has to do everything she can not to vomit, chewing the insides of her cheeks until the smell eventually fades into the background.

The worst part of the sickness has been the lack of a diagnosis. She'd be happy if they told her it was cancer: then at least she would know what she was dealing with. Instead, they mumble words like: nonspecific, localised, abdominal MUS. None of it means anything. The only thing that means something is her tolerance for pain. They don't need to give her the hard stuff, because they know she can take it.

In the meantime, she worries she is dying.

The university had a mental health and wellbeing officer. After months of sleepless nights, desperation drew her towards his office like a lamb to the slaughter. Immediately, his demeanour made her insides recoil: this was not right; it didn't feel right. But convention forced her bottom onto his chair – she couldn't turn around now she had entered, obviously. She sat there, glued to its hard seat, and imagined she was made of stone. Nothing came out.

We have an appointment, he said.

She commanded her head to move up, down.

Why are you here to see me? he tried again. And this time, his voice was infected with something like exasperation, or maybe boredom. It didn't encourage her to speak. There was something about the way his eyes were roving over her face, her hair(?), her clothes, that made her want to scream out. But she couldn't say anything, still.

172

OK, he said. OK. I've got here in my notes – and his eyes flicked towards his desk crowded with papers and two empty coffee mugs and a picture frame facing him – you're not sleeping well. That you're feeling quite anxious?

He didn't need to say anything more for her to know that he wasn't going to help her. She wanted to run out of the office at that very moment, but her legs were not listening to her brain's commands.

Listen, he said. Most people feel anxious because they're not prepared enough. Now I don't know what it was like for you at school, but university is different, yeah? You should pay attention in class, take notes, study. If you know what you're talking about, maybe you'll feel less anxious, eh?

He leaned back, satisfied that he had said something of value, and looked at her expectantly. She couldn't bear it.

Thank you, she whispered and leapt out of the chair and out of the room and out of the university grounds. She wanted nothing more in that moment than to cease to exist. This is the trigger of her illness: her body telling her stubborn mind to stop; saying no: we can't do this any more.

If it was possible to catalogue all of the things that had led her to this moment, she thinks she would have a fair shot of doing so. Her life split neatly into two parts – there was her life before university, and her life afterwards.

In part i, the defining moment was the raid. No, more specifically than that: it was the revulsion in the officer's voice when she barked at her mother to *speak English*. It was the sharp jolt of realisation that they were different and dirty for it, as she was recompensed for spying through the crack of the door and out onto a mess that was only ever meant to be witnessed by those who were older than her. It was the look on her mother's face, sweat rolling down her temples and gathering in the furrows of her eyes, arms cruelly held behind her back with her wrists encased in metal: *I'm sorry*.

Every time there's an unannounced visitor, an unexpected rap on the door, she gets palpitations.

In part ii, there is no defining moment. Rather, it is a series of moments.

She wanted so badly to please them. To make them proud. Remember: she was representing a *nation*, not just one family. And she wanted to remedy the flaw in her design: that she was born in Nigeria – whether happenstance or fate, it corrupted her existence in this country, and required her to prove herself. Every application to the Home Office meticulously detailed her grades. She is a good student. See, officers? She adds *value*.

Part iii is now: the ending.

She remembers the first time she learned to hate Rosy. The sweet little girl in whose hair she would bury her nose just to inhale the smell of her; her little companion, whose cheeks, even now, never lost their baby-like fullness.

Rosy was eleven and she was going to France with her class.

Rosy did not need a visa to travel.

Rosy had a British passport, and a strong south London accent, and – even at the tender age of eleven – a quiet self-assuredness that you couldn't fake.

Envy rose like bile in the back of her throat. She knew she was supposed to be happy for Rosy, and she wanted to be but she couldn't do it. It was hard to see past the fact that Rosy looked like her and came from a similar household, but Rosy was going to France with her school, and she most certainly was not.

Rosy's shadow wasn't heavy. It didn't try to envelop her into its arms and compress her with a unique gravitational pull. Rosy's shadow was a light-footed companion; a friend appearing only on sunny days. Rosy bounced like light refracted from moment to moment as her life fell into place. Then there she herself was. She bore her shadow like a cross, while she continued to endure the unholy matrimony that bound her to existence.

When the chance to reinvent herself arose, she grabbed it with desperate heat. She'd long since moulded her vowels to match theirs (unlike Rosy, who was allowed to heedlessly continue with her south London melody). Her hair was pulled back into a low bun, after paying £59 to have it relaxed: braids would not do, and an afro was out of the question, of course. Annoyingly, bits kept escaping, the September drizzle causing it to rise buoyantly and irresistibly above her hairline. And she couldn't quite rid herself of the smell of the hair cream she'd applied to keep it at bay. Even though she'd lathered herself in Coco Chanel, these were the tell-tale giveaways that identified her.

It seems stupid now, when she looks back on it, that she had thought that wearing a floral yellow cardigan would disguise her. They all muscled into the lecture theatre, the atmosphere a recognisably distinct mixture of the nerves and excitement of first-year students. She didn't know anyone, and she didn't know where to sit.

At the end of the lecture, the professor asked a question about the meaning of economics. This was the moment. She wanted to be noticed in a good way for once, and she took it. Steeling herself, she raised her hand, and answered.

People in the lecture theatre craned their necks round to

look at who had had the confidence to answer a question on the very first day, and she felt the blood rising to her cheeks and wondered if she'd made a terrible mistake.

Very good, came the response, and she wanted to die of pride.

On the way out of the lecture theatre, one of the boys who had been sitting a few rows ahead of her gave her a gentle slap on the back.

Nice one, mate, he said, his blue eyes literally twinkling in the LEDs of the hall. She willed her face not to betray her mind, which was suddenly tortured with images of herself lounging with this boy and his friends at his country house in the summer. I thought you'd be a roadman! And he laughed and walked out of the room with his friends.

She sat down on an empty seat and stayed there until the entire theatre had emptied, and then for another twenty minutes after that.

Alcohol was a fiery magic that ripped through her throat and burst out of her chest like a big shiny badge of confidence. They welcomed her willingness to participate with wide open arms – she could be one of them when her tongue was loose and her body was limber. But really, it made no sense because the drunk version of her was not really her at all.

The first time she seriously contemplated death was about fifteen shots in. Quite startlingly, past the sheen of ten sickly-sweet VKs and twerking on a sticky club floor, she knew that this – what they loved – wasn't her. It filled her with a despair so vast and unexpected that she staggered to the floor. Someone laughed and helped her to her feet – one too many drinks, love? – and she suddenly felt completely alone. The people around her repulsed her. She repulsed herself. She tore out of the club, promptly threw up on the pavement and sat there sobbing and hiccupping until it felt like her body had broken in two.

Don't you know she doesn't live with her parents? She lives with her cousins because her mum's been arrested and her dad ran away from the police. The *immigration* police.

For some reason, words had always stayed with her. Memory is supposed to be like springy green grass. You need to go over it again and again and again until a path is trodden. That's why she spent sunny days locked in her room with a pen and paper, a stack of books like a tower. She went over and over the words so she couldn't forget. So one day, she could make them proud. So she could represent her nation. Her generation.

But for some reason, words stayed with her. Her memory had no green grass. It was dry, brittle earth. Each word caused a fissure so deep it almost reached the lava of her.

She's annoyed at the fact that the memory that has returned to her in this moment is the one of the party. She doesn't want to remember that right now. She wants memories of Rosy in their childhood, she wants the taste of green mango reminding her of something distant but familiar, she wants the time before it all began.

But the stupid party is replaying in her mind. The way Sophie had said: No, it's because you're black.

They were so young; her hair not wanting anything to do with being yanked into submission, desperately trying to escape the twists, with the blackness of her scalp exposed (yes, even her insides were black). Sophie's hair was as slippery as a fish, hanging limply around her shoulders and shining like spun gold. Sophie was dewy. Next to her, she felt impalpable and repugnant. And yet – somehow still – they were friends.

It was Sophie's father who said no blacks at your party, honey. What he really meant was no immigrants. Sophie told her this matter-of-factly; at the age of eight, there is no sheepish grimace to convey a guilty relief at the fact there is somebody else to blame. There are only facts. It's as simple as black and white.

She was born in Nigeria, but she does not feel Nigerian. She lives in England, but she has thus far managed to avoid becoming British.

What does it feel like to own somewhere? To lay claim to a place as your home because your family have been there for generations? To know the soil as if you are made of its clay? To have your identity mapped into its line? To have your family tree's roots dug so deep into the ground that removal would threaten the very foundations of the earth?

She remembers thinking that she thought London would be clean. Even her five-year-old mind had an impression of the country of her ancestors' colonisers – unblemished and shiny.

She'd heard of London Bridge (falling down) and the London Eye. She didn't envisage that there were places like Catford, where amidst all the concrete, in the corners and the cracks, gatherings of plastic bags lurked, black with London grime instead of red with iron dust.

No different to Lagos, then, other than the colour of the dirt.

It is at university that she realises why her mum didn't want her catching the Tube alone, at the tender age of fourteen, wary of all the paedos. She catches herself staring at a girl with feline features; a little upturned nose and a tumble of silk for hair.

She wants to look away but she can't stop absorbing every

one of her features and wondering what it would be like to possess her.

There had been a time when she had possessed another woman. And when it was over – well and truly over – the pain felt warranted: her just deserts for breaking God's sacred code. Love, whose vigour had once pumped through her with the wild abandon of youth, had left her for good; loneliness now danced around her mockingly, encasing her chest in its vice-like embrace. So this was grief: remembering and regretting. The desire to snatch back a moment, to rewind time into a space where their hands were still entangled and their breath still shared the same air.

In moments like these, it was impossible to turn to God: you can't ask for help when the source of your pain is your sin.

Six years old
   Tracing the words on the pages of the Bible
   Paper so thin it seemed to dissolve beneath her fingers
   She was almost scared to touch it
   For some reason she felt that she could confide in God.

The first heartbreak she learned was from Auntie June. A woman who took summer's name, and embodied summer's spirit, who smelt like a buttery peach crumble and who was closer to her than her own mother. But even Auntie June didn't understand that a child of five can have feelings that are greater than their whole world.

When Auntie June found the Bible, she grabbed her arm so tightly that it felt like a Chinese burn. Delivered in the fierce, quiet whisper of a pastor's wife: Why would you write this? If you do this – people will forget you.

*If your hand causes you to sin, cut it off. If your foot causes you to sin, cut it off. And if your eye causes you to sin, tear it out.* What if your mind causes you to sin, Auntie June? What do you do then?

Her eyes are not open, but she can tell that there are people coming in and out of the room; doctors scurry around her, nurses prod and poke her arms. Unfamiliar voices. Did they not tell anyone at home? She squeezes her eyes but can't stop the tears from dribbling out the sides. She's alive. It surprises her and annoys her that, after everything, she wants to live.

# In the Belly of the Flask

## Franki Ayres

### As told to Rebecca Pert

Where did it begin?

I think back, as far as I can, to my first food. My mother's amniotic fluid. They say flavours filter through in the womb; garlic, aniseed, carrot, mint, gulped down in the warm, sloshing darkness. Did my mum deny herself anything, did she lose her appetite? Is that why I developed a taste for lack, for absence? No, the only thing she couldn't stomach was caffeine. Tea and coffee. It was a cup of tea that gave me away, back in 1979, as she declined a cuppa in the kitchen of 14 Meadow Close.

'Are you pregnant?' asked my nan.

What does being afraid taste like? I wonder if it flavoured the water of her womb; sharp and metallic.

My mum wasn't supposed to be pregnant. I was a secret. She hid her swelling belly for as long as she could, wishing me smaller, shrunk, invisible. But she was happy to be pregnant, glowing with her secret knowledge, smiling above her concealing smock dresses.

She thought I was a boy. She had a hunch, an instinct, and she named me Daniel.

It's only now I realise that Daniel is an anagram of Denial.

After birth, a healthy baby, placed on the parent's belly or chest, will move instinctively towards the nipple to initiate feeding. Navigating by the scent of milk, the sound of voice, the touch of skin, the infant drags themselves towards their first meal, latches on, and begins to suckle. Each touch of the nipple provides a surge of oxytocin to parent and child, a flood of love in chemical form, sparkling across the synapses. The first milk, colostrum, is liquid gold; yellow in colour, thick and rich, full of fat, nutrients, antibodies.

But I am born too soon, after too long a labour, my oxygen compromised.

'Go with her!' Mum cries to my dad as I am rushed to the neonatal unit, to an incubator, a plastic tank. How am I fed? Through a tube, through a drip, through a bottle? Nobody seems to know. My dad is ushered out of the room. My first meal, shrouded in mystery; eating already a complicated thing.

As a child, sensations – textures, smells, tastes and temperatures – affect me in strange ways. Perhaps there is a jumbled connection somewhere in my brain, a rogue synaptic pathway. Things that other children do effortlessly, thoughtlessly – eat buttered toast, wear hairbands, pull up long socks – make my skin cringe. I wince at surfaces that feel slick, greasy, slithery, smooth. I dislike the looseness of skirts floating against my legs; I hate the knee-high white socks we wear to school in summer, their lacy pattern peppered with tiny holes. After I button my school shirt my fingertips feel sullied; I want to spit out their taste. I wear my winter uniform all through spring and into summer, sweating in my heavy brown skirt, my thick tights,

182

rather than feel the slithery kisses of breeze and cotton against bare thigh. I watch the boys in their grey trousers with envy.

At mealtimes my throat closes against the stringy texture of meat-pie chunks, the plasticky brittleness of choc ices. I chew and chew, unable to swallow, until eventually I spit the mush into a tissue.

'Fussy', my parents call me. Ironic, for someone who hates fuss and froth and frill, who finds relief in matte textures, coarse fabrics, dry bread. My dad sits me down and tells me to write a list of foods that *for God's sake, you will eat.*

I only eat two types of sandwich: Marmite, or strong yellow cheese. Both have to be constructed of brown bread, with absolutely no butter or margarine. My dad makes my lunches the night before, at the same time as his own, wrapping the sandwiches in kitchen roll and stowing them neatly in my lunchbox.

I love my lunchbox. It is large and red and rectangular, with a matte hatched texture that I like to run my fingers over. Two huge clips secure the contents with a deep, satisfying click. But best of all is the sticker scene on the front: Darth Vader, cloak flaring behind him, flanked by two armed Stormtroopers against a snowy backdrop of twisted silver trees. I have a matching flask, too, on which Darth Vader stands with his arms crossed, an image of black-caped confidence.

The dinner ladies supervise us at lunchtime, chivvying us along.

'Make sure you eat all your crusts,' they say. 'It'll make your hair curly.'

Slowly, the children finish their lunches and empty out onto the playground. I end up rounded onto the table with the other dawdlers, the slow chewers, the daydreamers. But I have a magic trick. A vanishing act, Darth Vader my assistant. What I will not, cannot eat, he consumes for me, bread and cheese stuffed surreptitiously into the belly of the flask, safely guarded behind his crossed arms.

I lift my lunchbox up, clean but for a few persuading crumbs, to a dinner lady's impressed eye. I am waved on out to playtime, and I am free.

Young children don't tend to deny themselves anything, given the chance. They are pleasure seekers, a ball of impulse.

And yet, here I am, Easter come and gone, my chocolate eggs still untouched. Foil wrapped, box sealed, glinting dully on the shelf. My brother and sister eye them with bafflement, their own eggs long gone, torn into and devoured instantly.

A game, played only with myself – how long can I resist them? A day, two, three? The days tick by, the weeks, the months.

One year later, and still the eggs sit, gleaming on the shelf like saintly relics in a church. Their cool smooth wholeness, unbroken and pure, a symbol of my self-control, satisfies me in a way food itself does not.

To be a child is to be powerless, helpless, less than human. Things are done to you, rather than by you. The world is run by adults with their inscrutable rules and routines, their commands and queues and bells and punishments, mealtimes and bedtimes and bathtimes. Brush your teeth, open wide, eat your crusts, take your elbows off the table, speak up, pipe down, don't dawdle, don't cry, don't be silly. But I was learning these small acts of resistance, of denial – the closed mouth, the clenched teeth, the sandwich stuffed in a plastic flask, the chocolate eggs left unbroken – could hold power. Could give me something, some pocket of space that was all mine.

My parents consider my fussiness around food quirky, tiresome – infuriating, even, but there is no real concern, no alarm. I am a skinny kid, but then so was my mum; she was teased in the playground, as I am: she was 'Olive Oyl', 'bony maloney', 'skinny as a stick of macaroni'; I am 'skinny malinky', 'lanky', 'chicken legs'. She laughed off her insults, she laughs off mine, she defends my body to me. My slimness, to her, is familiar, is normal, more so than my sister's body, which has always been naturally rounder and softer – adorable baby rolls morphing into pre-teen puppy fat.

To other adults, however, my slimness is not normal. At Brownies – already a chore; I feel stupid dancing around a toadstool and would far rather be at Cubs with my brother – Tawny Owl takes the piece of string from the brown leather pouch on my belt and wraps it twice around my waist, marvelling at how thin I am. My cheeks burn. When I get home, I tell my mum. I tell her how upset I am. I tell her I don't want to go to Brownies any more.

What I don't tell her is the secret, confusing gratification I felt; the shiver of pleasure that came from my body being remarkable, being *special*.

What she doesn't know, can't know, is that *her* skinny is not *my* skinny.

I am eleven years old and I am crammed into a cupboard, the door closed, hot with righteous anger. I have decided that non-human beings have the right to life as much as Homo sapiens. I am horrified by the idea of the abattoir, the bolt through the brain, the chopping block; by the idea of taking a life to make a meal, of eating corpse-flesh that once had eyes to see me. I have the courage of my convictions, I am as fervent as a martyr, and I am refusing to leave the cupboard until my parents agree that I can be a vegetarian.

'All right,' they sigh. 'Fine.'

I emerge from the cupboard, cramp-limbed, feeling lighter. The list of foods I will eat has shrunk even smaller. But now, at least, to my parents' relief, there are clear rules to follow, some logic behind the fussiness. Linda McCartney becomes a staple of my diet. Every meal now tastes of dehydrated soya, whatever meat it is supposed to be. The consistency, of taste and texture, makes things easier for me. It is a food I can trust.

The battles around the dinner table become fewer. And my disordered eating finds a new disguise, an acceptable public face.

My parents, I'm sure, think this is another fad, a phase that will be forgotten in a few days' time. But I know better. I have won again; another sly snatch of control.

And then something happens which I cannot control, no matter how hard I try, no matter how much I refuse. I cannot lock myself away in a cupboard from it, I cannot close my mouth against it, I cannot stuff it in a flask to be binned later.

Puberty.

Most of my classmates have already started their periods. I am certain it won't happen to me. It only happens to *real* girls, which I feel – have always felt, on some fundamental level – that I am not. I am not sure exactly what I *am*, not yet, but I relate more to the men in my family than the women. I am similar to them, in bone structure and body hair, in my thoughtful personality, in the way I talk with my hands. Furtively, in the bathroom, I practise shaving an imaginary beard, using my dad's Gillette foam and the handle of my plastic toothbrush as a cut-throat razor, gliding tracks across my frothy cheeks, pulling faces in the mirror – eyebrows raised, mouth puckered, upper lip stretched, relishing the minty tingle, the softness of the foam. I secretly love it when I'm mistaken for a boy, kicked out of ladies' toilets and changing rooms. 'She's a girl, stupid!' my brother spits, indignant, protective, as I stand by, glowing.

As more and more girls in my class get their periods, I relax.

It's not happening to me. My sheer force of will has kept it at bay. I can control it, I can say *no*.

And yet my body has other plans. Covertly, it has been sending messages, secret codes, between the hypothalamus, the pituitary gland, the ovaries – and, inevitably, one day, it comes.

It isn't dramatic. It isn't even that bloody. It is a deep, aching menstrual pain that hits my stomach with a punch. It is nausea lingering long after I flush the browned tissue away. It is the cotton sanitary pad my mum gives me, inches thick, wedge-shaped, that feels grotesque, invasive, stuffed between my legs.

I spend the day curled up on my younger sister's bed, on her pink and purple duvet, surrounded by her teddies; seeking comfort in this prepubescent space, perhaps – a sanctuary of childhood. I clutch her stuffed toys. I cry into their fur. I wish that I was one of them; inanimate and bloodless.

But my body keeps changing. Overnight, it seems, it stretches and swells and softens in ways that feel revolting. The touch of my flesh against itself is so unkind. Breasts rest against my ribs, and on a hot day the sweat trapped in these small crevices feels excessive, grotesquely slippery. Running, dancing, even walking, these soft lumps on my chest move in their own nauseating rhythm, grasping onto my skin, parasitic. I cannot stand the idea of a bra, soft lace cupping and caring for this unwelcome flesh. I stuff the lumps instead into undersized sports tops; I squash them as flat as possible.

I want to be square-edged, hard, angular; as free in my body as the boys seem to be, as my older brother is. We were so close. But now our roads diverge; I am careening down a separate track, a track that leads to womanhood, and I hate it. I want to get back to where I was before, whittle my new body away, starve off the round edges, pare myself down, down, as far as my bones, hard and clean and sexless.

The Conservatives brought in Section 28 – the local govern-ment act that banned local authorities and schools from 'promoting homosexuality' – when I was nine years old. So, as I navigate my adolescence, there are no books, no films, no discussions, no affirmative education around same-sex rela-tionships. Homophobia at school is rife. Being gay or lesbian is something to ridicule, something disgusting, something to be feared.

My route to school involves crossing a dual carriageway through an underpass. There, spray-painted on the walls, are hateful homophobic slurs. They name one of my brother's friends, my favourite one, a kind, friendly, chatty boy who sits at our kitchen table and talks to my mum and me about photography and bikes. I have an intense crush on him. I fanta-sise about him being my friend too, one day, when I'm older. Maybe more than a friend.

But one day he vanishes. He has moved away from the area, for his own safety, to escape the violence. I am bereft. I am furious.

There is fear and stigma around HIV and AIDS. One day a visiting minister – part of a Christian group which arrives on a bus each year – tells my sister's classmates that these are diseases created by God to wipe out homosexuals. My sister tells me what he said, and I storm the bus, burning with anger, to confront him. I am disciplined by the school for my outburst. But not by my parents.

My mum and dad are open-minded people. They ignore Section 28 whenever discussions around sexuality come up in their workplaces, although they don't bring up the subject at home. I can't talk to them about my own feelings, my confusion around gender, my burgeoning sexuality. For a start, there is no language for how I am feeling, this deep discomfort. How can I describe something which has no words?

Secondly, I'm not sure how much they really understand. They know about love, but the practicalities of gay sex? Of sexual health, of safety?

But mostly, I can't risk losing them. When the outside world is so hate-filled, when love is so uncertain, I'm not ready to jeopardise any of their love for me. How can I know, for sure, that their acceptance of others' differences will extend to me? It's one thing to chat with your son's gay friend at your kitchen table, but when your own child tells you they're queer?

Decades later, when I tell my mum that I've changed my pronouns, she tells me that gender doesn't matter to her. When I'm a teenager, she makes similar comments about sexuality. I understand that what she wants her children to know is that we are loved unconditionally. But what I cannot express, growing up, is the feeling of distance, the knowledge that she loves me from the safety of being heterosexual and cisgendered.

I don't want to have to explain. I want them to just *know*. But that isn't possible. So, instead, I stay silent.

In my wallet I carry a piece of paper, on which is the number for the Lesbian and Gay Switchboard. Occasionally I slide into a phone box, unfold the paper, lift the receiver – but I always find a reason why this is not the right phone box, not this time, not yet. Over time, I fold and unfold the paper so much that the numbers wear away from the page.

But there is one place. One sanctuary, one space that offers relief, recognition, safety. I take Drama for GCSE. The department is run by a brilliant heterosexual surrealist couple. They open my world, expand my horizons, share with me the work of diverse theatre companies, led by queer bodies, black and brown bodies, disabled bodies. I begin to see people like me looking back at me.

One day we are shown a video, a piece of physical theatre

entitled *Enter Achilles* by a company called DV8. Eight men in a smoky pub, gathered around a jukebox. Through movement and dance the performers explore masculinity and queerness, their bodies telling a story of pain, desire, transgression. It compels me, it scares me; it feels risky, sensual, watching these men dance dangerously, clutching their pints of beer, their cigarettes.

I begin to spend all my lunchtimes in the small black theatre space, in front of the square TV on its big trolley, watching, rewinding, re-watching the video. I barely breathe, my mouth dry with desire. I want to be one of those half-naked men, falling into the arms of another, clasping hands, lifting hips, rolling over bodies, over tables, over the floor, coming closer to the lens – where I sit on the other side watching, avidly studying their positions, their expressions, their gestures.

My best friend joins me. She loves the performance as much as I do, although for different reasons. We act out the scene together, watching, rehearsing, re-watching, rehearsing. I practise and practise until I become one of those men, moving my own body the way they move theirs.

Alongside this eruption of desire comes an eruption of discomfort with my body, more vicious even than in puberty. When I start having sex, removing the layers of clothing that conceal the soft growths on my chest, always so much larger than my lovers expect, I feel so ashamed. It is as if my nakedness, instead of being my truth, my most raw state, is a costume; an ill-fitting outfit I can't take off.

I seek a double mastectomy on the NHS. My breasts are physically, painfully, weightily intolerable, it's true. But this isn't *the* truth. I need parts of me removing in order to feel whole.

I am photographed by a stranger, naked from the waist up, from five different angles, the pictures sent to a panel of 'expert' decision-makers to scrutinise. Am I worthy? Will they fund my mastectomy?

The answer is a decisive no.

My hatred towards my body continues to grow. I eat less and less, I stop nourishing it. Before going out dancing, before having sex, I cannot eat. I need to feel empty.

If anybody is going to touch my body, I want there to be nothing for them to find.

I am twenty-two years old and I am in pain.

Investigations – blood tests, X-rays, MRI scans – rule out viruses, cancers, injuries, rheumatoid arthritis, ankylosing spondylitis. Each torn-up diagnosis is a relief, and a source of frustration. What is it, what's wrong with me? Why do I ache, why do I burn, why does a caress from a partner, or the weight of my favourite wool coat, hurt me so much?

The list of potential ailments shrinks and shrinks until there is only one left: fibromyalgia.

My nerves are short-circuiting. Like a faulty fire alarm, stuck beeping shrilly in a smokeless house, my wiry, overexcitable body can interpret any sensation as pain, shooting an urgent danger signal to my brain even when nothing is wrong.

I am sent to a pain management clinic – is there a more dispiriting phrase than 'pain management'? – and sit in a room with other people in pain, incurable pain, unendurable pain, all clutching our X-rays and scans and reports, wanting answers that we know we're not going to get. At this point in my life, it is the most depressing room I have ever been in.

'We are here to help you cope,' the doctors and therapists assure us. And then they tell us that the programme will not be starting for another six to eight months.

I go home. I plummet. Within a couple of weeks I am prescribed my first antidepressants.

This can't be the end of the road. It can't be. I cannot accept it. I will not. I launch myself into finding a solution, anything that will cure me, that will give me a moment's respite from the perpetual flu-like aching, the sharp stabbing and spasming, the gnaw, the tingle, the sting, the burn. Osteopathy, acupuncture, yoga therapy, meditation, TENS machines, hot baths, heat pads, painkillers, cannabis, CBD, muscle relaxants, memory foam mattresses, supportive shoes. I develop scars in places where the pain is most persistent from the boiling hot-water bottles I press directly into my flesh, a pain that *I* can control. *Here, brain*, I think, as I sear my skin. *This is for you.* I blow money that I do not have, burning through multiple overdrafts on my quest for pain relief; I travel to Goa to study t'ai chi, I visit a shaman who lays me down on a darkly oiled piece of tree wood and pummels my body until I hallucinate, until I am sick. I swim in the sea and feel weightless and cradled, as I must have done as a foetus in the womb. I wish I could go back to that black unknowingness. I do not want to feel any more of me.

And then I discover literature on fibromyalgia and food. A strict diet, I read, can help. I research, intensively, making scores of notes and charts and lists. Eliminating some foods can soothe the pain, while eating others will hurt me. Processed food is out. Additives are out. Gluten is out. Caffeine is out. Fresh fruit is good, but only if it's organic and not in the nightshade family. A vegetarian diet is good, vegan even better. Some books are vague, discussing toxins and impurities, while others are scientific, talking about oxidative stress, arachidonic acid, beta-carotene, resveratrol, polyphenols. Down the rabbit hole I fall, clutching desperately to the books' motivational exhortations: *You have the power to heal yourself. Take responsibility for your health. Own it! Unleash it! Reclaim it!*

The list of foods I can eat shrinks and shrinks. My cupboards begin to look like a health food shop. And yet my gut starts to feel sluggish, sore, irritable. I don't realise, yet, that these are signs of starvation. I am obviously eating the wrong foods, I think, inflaming my insides, letting toxins into my system. I turn to yet another diet, the candida diet, and the lists shrink further. Fruits are out. Rice is out. Yeast is out.

I have also been visiting an Ayurvedic doctor. I am prescribed a *Vata* diet. I'm told it will help with pain, cramps, tension, bloating, anxiety, constipation, dryness. I'm told to eat small quantities. I'm told not to eat to fullness. I'm told to fast regularly. I write down a list: FOODS TO AVOID, a full page of scribbled details. On the opposite page, FOODS TO INCREASE is left blank.

My 'fussy' childhood restrictions look laughable now. I no longer eat dry bread, Marmite, hard yellow cheese. I now eat the bones of food, the ghosts of food: tablets, capsules, powders, protein mixes, vitamin supplements. At one point the only thing I will consume is water in which quinoa has briefly soaked. And yet, strangely, I am drawn to food. Like checking on my clutch of silvery eggs and seeing them whole and untouched, it gives me a sense of fulfilment to scour the supermarket shelves, scrutinising all the packets and tins and jars, reciting the ingredients in my head, calculating the breakdown of energy: fat, carbs, protein, fibre, sugars; listing mentally all the reasons why I cannot consume them.

This can last hours.

Is it possible to become attached to non-attachment? To become addicted to giving things up?

When I leave the shop I feel full up on emptiness.

I don't recognise that I have anorexia. Other people don't, either. It is a manipulative and secret illness, and pulls the wool over everyone's eyes, including my own.

It's easy to hide. I live alone. I wear baggy clothes, layers of them, an attempt to keep out the cold along with any suspicion. I eat occasionally at social events; I don't allow anyone to see me naked.

It's not that people don't recognise my frailty – I have widespread musculoskeletal pain accompanied by fatigue, poor sleep, memory and mood difficulty – but I blame these on my fibromyalgia. Anorexia hides in plain sight.

I collect other people's behaviours, their methods, their systems to lose weight, informing anyone close by that I need to know this method to help me 'maintain'.

Soon I begin to follow not just my own rules around food, but others' also.

I am an addict, and the addiction and starvation have changed the physiology of my brain, altering the circuitry so fundamentally that I feel I am doing all I can to survive, even while I am starving myself to death.

Ten years pass. Ten years in which I barely manage to cling on. I lose everything: my work, my partner, my home. My desire to live. I lurch between crises, supported by my auntie, her warm hands caring for me, until eventually even she accepts that I am beyond her help. I am admitted to hospitals, to psychiatric wards, where my body is treated – stabilised, at least, although my bones continue to crumble, and my heart continues to weaken, its pulse fluttering erratically, a butterfly with a torn wing – but my mind, my soul, are still starving.

Even as I am admitted into a specialist NHS eating disorder unit, I am still trying to negotiate. Still trying to say *no*. My auntie is with me, and I try to get her to agree that I don't need to be there. But she holds firm. She tells me that this place will give my body the best chance to live.

'Give it your best shot,' she says. 'Really *try*.'

In the unit there is no negotiating. No bargains, no tricks. I will eat. It will be incremental, in tune with daily blood tests to avoid refeeding syndrome – the potentially fatal shift in fluid and electrolytes that can happen when a starving person begins to eat – but I *will* eat, and I will eat all the foods I have not eaten in months, years, decades, in a relatively short space of time.

As if I have time-travelled back to the beginning, back to being a baby in an incubator, my first food is milk. 250 ml of warm, whole, cow's milk. I am told soy milk is an option, but I'll have to drink double the quantity. I am horrified.

I ask to see the dietician. She listens, sympathetically, to my anxious pleas, but she won't relent. 'I suggest you eat and drink the food recommended,' she tells me. 'Trust us to help you by making the choices *for* you.'

The unit's dining room smells just like the school canteen. Boiled vegetables, mop water, dishwasher steam. But instead of dinner ladies there are nurses and healthcare assistants, and instead of sandwich crusts I must consume Ensure: a bastard version of colostrum; a nutrient-dense, calorie-packed 'milk-shake'; liquid beige rather than liquid gold. Its ingredients include such inscrutable things as choline chloride, calcium pantothenate and potassium phosphate dibasic, and it comes in several flavours: banana, vanilla, fruits of the forest, peach, coffee and 'neutral'.

Ensure is what we are given if we don't eat our 'real' food. Even one bite left on our plate merits an entire bottle. It is served chilled, glopped into mugs, a clear plastic straw popped in. Most of the mugs have the eating disorder unit's logo emblazoned on the side, but some are speckled with flaking paint; decorated a few months ago by an occupational therapy group, scoured by repeated dishwasher cycles into an abstract mess of colour.

I do not have Darth Vader, now, but his crossed-arm confidence, the magic tricks, remain.

The nurse pours the Ensure into the mug, adds a straw — and then makes the mistake of turning her back to me. In one swift swipe I grab the empty bottle and pour the shake back into it. I present the empty mug to the nurse, and am let out — not to a playground, this time, but to the supervised lounge, the bottle hidden deep in my pocket, heavy with its sticky secret.

But eating disorder staff are sharper to tricks than dinner ladies. My ruse works for a week or two, baffling the nurses. Why am I not gaining weight? I am smug, I am sly — but I get cocky and casual. Perhaps, subconsciously, I sabotage myself — the other patients are on to me, of course, and the guilt is gnawing at me.

One day a healthcare assistant spots me mid-pour. Disaster. He makes me stand up and hand it over, then goes to the kitchen and gets a new shake. Opens it, pours the contents into a fresh mug, places it in front of me. Sits down opposite me. Watches.

No way out. No tricks, no ruses, no Darth Vader. I sit there staring at the mug, the beige liquid. Slowly, almost everyone around me finishes their lunches, their puddings, their Ensures, and begins ordering coffee or peppermint tea to take into the lounge — the reward for those who eat everything and finish on time. I am left alone, with this man and his hateful milkshake.

He tries a few tired methods — cajoling, being funny, being angry. I don't have to try to be angry; I'm furious, with him and with myself. I feel stuck, powerless, paralysed, a helpless child once more, caught between two forces, one shouting *Yes* and the other shouting *No*, their strength equal, unbearable, making me boil. A wave of blistering fury sweeps through my body and before I know what I'm doing I stand up, grab the mug, raise my arm, intending to throw it at him, *hard* — but then, just as quickly, I reverse my aim and tip the shake over my head.

The glop splatters onto my hair. Gloops down my face, onto my shoulders, my sleeves.

I drop the mug. The HCA and I stare at each other, both shocked. He doesn't laugh, although it's ridiculous, *I* look ridiculous, the sticky beige liquid dripping off my nose, onto my slippers. I start to cry.

He doesn't try to stop me as I walk out of the dining room. I go down the corridor and into my room, lie down on the bed, curl up into my jumper, still covered in the sticky sickly shake.

I am worn out, I am in pain, and this has only just begun. In about two hours' time, there will be another Ensure waiting for me in the same dining room.

I can't pull the wool over anyone's eyes any more. My friends and family know, now, how sick I am. They are scared, they are confused. They are angry.

'Just EAT!' they say.

How can someone from the outside understand how something so simple, so natural, could be so impossible? How drinking a glass of milk could feel like drinking arsenic? How could they understand how starting feels like giving up? How I am trying to save my life by starving myself?

'How can you do this to our family? You don't love us. You love anorexia more.'

This hurts more than anything to hear. How can I begin to explain? None of us *choose* this. Look, I want to say, come in the dining room with me, see these two mums, both eating six times a day, through tears, silent raging internal battles, forcing down food, with a photo of their kids in front of them, desperately fighting to get home. How can anyone say these parents do not love their children? That they love anorexia more?

197

'I will not share you with anorexia. I refuse to collaborate with anorexia.'

My oldest, most loyal friend – the girl who shared my lunchtime drama rehearsals – tells me this. She has to step away from me, to protect herself, to protect her young son from my illness. I am dying, and she is scared. I respect that. I understand it. She never leaves me emotionally – we write to each other – but she cannot be near me physically.

But I form new bonds, in hospital. Friendships amongst patients are forged swiftly and fiercely. After all, we often understand each other far better than our family and friends on the 'outside' do.

We have our own bonding rituals. Knitting is one. One of the patients is a fashion student. He teaches another how to knit, and it soon becomes a trend, wonky scarves sprouting and spreading across laps, the click-click of needles a percussive undercurrent to the noise of daytime TV. Cross-stitch is another, the meditative punching and threading. We tend to each other through touch: shoulder massages, nail painting, makeup application, hair styling. I even allow some of this to be done to me, my straggly curls straightened, worn this way for a week or so. We ask the staff to grant us weekly film nights, and these become a ritual too; we savour our allocated warm drink in the communal lounge, in the pyjamas gifted to us by the staff at Christmas, and watch movies: Disney films, psychological horrors, slasher flicks.

But friendships in hospital are as cryptic and slippery as our illnesses are. We show each other kindness, empathy, love. We encourage each other to eat because we care about each other. We believe in each other's lives. We want each other to be free from suffering.

But we also encourage each other to eat because we want to 'win'.

Anorexia poisons everything pure; it twists and taints and sours.

What does 'winning' look like? I don't know. There is no end goal here – no logical one, anyway. Anorexia kills. It has the highest mortality rate of any psychiatric illness. Half the time it kills through medical complications brought about by starvation. The other half of the time, it kills by suicide. This is the endgame. This is the prize we 'win'.

Treatment for anorexia is about 'returning'. Returning to your family, children, siblings, parents, friends. To college, to university, to work. Returning to yourself.

But what if you don't want to return to yourself?

What if, instead, you want to transform?

I have a new therapist. I like her a lot. She is tiny; when she pokes her head round the large white door of my bedroom, smiling, I'm always struck by how small she looks. I follow her quick, soft footsteps down the corridor to our therapy room. The space is clinical, with an unfriendly plastic sofa, but she warms it somehow, with her deeply coloured dresses, her kind brown eyes.

It is in these sessions that things truly begin to change.

She runs group therapy sessions, too. She uses Tarot cards, sometimes; round ones, illustrated by a friend, with beautifully inked designs. She throws them in the air so that they land, scattered, on the lounge floor, and we're encouraged to look at them, to take our time, and to pick up any that we are drawn to. The images work as a way of unlocking our thoughts, our emotions. Why did we choose the cards we did? We take it in turns to talk, until we are ready to stop. We listen to each other, with no objective. We offer no solutions, no comebacks, no reprimands. We listen, quietly. That is all. These sessions become one of the most healing spaces in my entire time as an inpatient.

'Our conversation reminds me of another patient I worked with about ten years ago,' my therapist tells me in a session one day. 'They were talking like you are, but we didn't have the language for it. I think perhaps they were transgender too.'

'What happened to them?' I ask.

'I don't know – I think, for them, their way of coping was to not talk about it.'

So, instead, we talk about it. There is language now for what I want, a name for the discomfort I feel in my core.

I feel lucky to work with this therapist. I also feel lucky that she is honest enough to know when I need more than she can offer.

She refers me to psychosexual therapy sessions, provided by another service. During these, I begin to unpack what has been underpinning a large part of my need for anorexia for so long.

It's not easy, or without conflict. I am still living in an environment with a programme heavily focused on body dysmorphia, and a treatment model whose aim is acceptance of my body, rather than a recognition of the need to change it. Staff tell me that I'm the first trans person they've ever treated, although I know that isn't true.

But I am supported. The clinic continues to provide a safe environment for me to push beyond medical stabilisation, to keep going, to bring my body to a healthy place, a place where I am well enough to undergo medical transition.

My therapist leaves before I am discharged. Before she goes, we have tea together. She has written me a letter.

'It has been a privilege to watch you fall a little more in love with the self you are becoming,' she writes, 'the self you are creating each week, and a self that is trying to "live into" the answers about his gender identity.'

Finally, I have been heard.

I make a quiet pact with myself to try and hang on to her words; to not lose hold of what she has seen in me.

'It has to start with food.' That is what everyone says. There are no shortcuts, no ways to skip to the end. To be well enough to receive transgender healthcare, I have to eat.

So, I eat. I eat my meals, my snacks, my Ensures. I begin to return to a person that is forced to appear 'well', maintaining my weight, trying my best to 'present' my gender identity in a body that is swelling, softening, feeling further and further away from my authentic self. My discomfort grows and gathers weight as my flesh does.

Again, my period arrives. I shouldn't be surprised. This is part of that plan. But still, there is terror as the familiar loss of control sweeps over me. My key nurse does not know what to do, beyond holding my hand and breathing with me through a panic attack.

I stop coming out of my room. I cannot be seen like this. Cards and notes are pushed under my door by worried patients, but I cannot reply to them, cannot explain what is happening. I am becoming increasingly distressed, unable to manage what is happening to my body.

'You have a fear of becoming a woman,' my consultant tells me one day, 'because you have a fear of becoming an adult.'

In some respects, she isn't wrong. The numb obsessiveness of anorexia has allowed me to avoid confronting feelings that have been locked away since childhood. But it is impossible for the consultant to see that her years of experience are narrowing, rather than expanding, her ability to listen. She is translating my feelings towards my changing body into a language she is more familiar with: that of a typical cisgendered female patient.

I ask to be referred to a gender identity clinic. Still the consultant presses pause.

201

The wait is too long, and the weight continues to go up. One day it is just too much.

I hate my body. I have eaten their disgusting food for ten months. I have worked hard in therapy, really *hard*, and for what? I am a child again, the adults stripping me of my power. I feel unsafe. I am angry. I want to hurt myself. I want to do something *to* my body that *I* have absolute control over. I want to say *fuck you*.

I take a craft knife and slash into my flesh, into my chest, into these soft hateful growths that are not a part of who I am, that are a symbol of powerlessness. I hate them, I hate them, I attack them and I don't know if I intend to strike as deep as I do – I'm not thinking, I'm not planning, I'm not in a space to think of any future, any consequences.

I return from A & E in the early hours and climb into bed. The hours tick by. I miss breakfast.

There is a knock at the door. A new locum doctor has arrived on the ward, and he asks if he can come in and sit with me a while, talk about what's happened.

I try, but I cannot find the words. As he leaves, he tells me that his door is always open.

My trust isn't immediate. I have been let down in the past. But gradually, as he takes care of my wounds over the coming weeks, we start to share. He shares his own queerness, and his experience working as a doctor within the queer community at large. It makes talking to him easier. I feel like I don't have to constantly advocate for myself, the way I do with other staff.

He isn't perfect, of course. But he is an ally. And one day, we sit together and write my first referral to a gender identity clinic.

'They can give you the help you need,' he tells me. 'The help you deserve.'

This gatekeeping entrance into trans healthcare still feels unnecessary, unfair. But at least he opens the gate for me. And he helps me to make peace somehow with my body, just enough to hold on to there being 'another way'.

A nurse removes the drains and dressings and binder and bandages which have been cocooning my chest post-surgery, in the August heatwave. A tight chrysalis. It splits open; I am released.

My friend, my loving witness, Vince, takes a photograph as I look into the hospital mirror.

I am two months away from forty, but the years have fallen away from my face. My expression is childlike, my eyes and smile wide. For the first time, since before my first puberty, I am seeing *myself*.

My chest is a straight line, down, steeply descending. I think of a cliff face, a rocky edge, eroded by a waterfall, a velocity cascading from a force somewhere inside me. Two fresh bilateral scars score my torso, neat puckered seams from the surgeon's knife. So different to the old white marks that lie on my skin. Despite the surgeon's skilful care in removing them, some still remain, a ghostly palimpsest, reminders of old hurt.

I am now forty-three years old.

Is this a happy ending? A tidy answer? Anorexia now cured?

Research tells us that fewer than half the people with this illness recover. 46 per cent of people will fully recover, 34 per cent improve partially, and 20 per cent develop chronic anorexia nervosa.

Which percentage do I fit into?

I want to tell you I'm in the 46 per cent, but I'm a realist by now. My body is still a battleground. I need to rest a lot. There are places I can't visit, things I can't do, my life circum-scribed by pain, by fatigue, by porous bones. Long-term malnutrition has taken its toll. The next steps in my medical transition are also compromised; there are difficult choices to be made. Nothing is simple for a body like mine. The impact of anorexia will continue to shape the rest of my life, and although I am hopeful, I can't pretend I don't get frightened.

What can tip the balance into despair is when the places I want to visit, the things that bring me purpose and connection to my community, are inaccessible; pointless, thoughtless barriers erected towards my disabled body. This distance, this shutting out, causes me anger, pain, resentment. It hurts me, and when it hurts, I am vulnerable to anorexia; I feel the lure of its clear, numb embrace.

It's uncomfortable for people to hear this, people who love me. But it's the truth.

I cannot promise this is a happy ending. But I can promise you that I do everything I can to try to nurture my body, which I have held on to with such effort, such difficulty. I do all the things I can to give myself the best chance of living. I am still in therapy. I'm not out of the woods yet, but I'm not in the densest trees any more.

I have found a way to be an artist again. Where once my sensitivities were deemed 'too much', they now inspire my work, and help me help others. And although my life can feel small, I live it big. I now listen differently, more carefully, more fully. I try to be present, fully present, in everything. I no longer want to leave the eggs on the shelf, gathering dust. I want to take them down, unpeel their foil, hold their convex ovoid curvature in my palm, the same size and shape as a human heart. I want to break off pieces and let them melt on my tongue. I may not ever be able to unthinkingly devour them. But I can still relish them. I can savour, and linger, and love.

Writing this chapter – with Rebecca's guiding touch – has

been a healing process, helping me to further understand my anorexia, to take another step in empowering my voice. Although this book describes the stories within as told by patients and service users, I don't think of myself like that. Patient comes from the Latin 'patiens', from 'patior', to suffer or bear. And whilst my story shares with you an experience of suffering, I am, deep down, who I have always been. I am the very same who reached out to others in hospital who were also in pain, who within their own suffering returned their love to me. I am not suffering, I am not bearing; this is not who we are.

Where am I now?

I think back, back to my very beginning. My mum was not wrong. I am not the gender I was assigned at birth. Daniel would perhaps have suited me, through childhood at least. A more comfortable name than the one I was given. But I am not Daniel, I'm Franki.

I'm not in denial. I am being frank. I'm telling the truth, with an open heart. Will you listen?

Franki. From Frank. A name of German origin.

It means 'a free man'.

If you or someone you know has been affected by any of the issues raised in this book, support is available and can be accessed via the resources below:

**NHS EVERY MIND MATTERS**
The centre for the NHS' mental health campaign, contains lots of guidance and support
https://www.nhs.uk/every-mind-matters/mental-health-issues/anxiety/

**MIND**
Supportive, reliable mental health information and services. Offer a network of local drop-in centres around England and Wales
Infoline 0300 123 3393
https://www.mind.org.uk/

**SAMARITANS**
Emotional support and suicide prevention
Free 24/7 helpline 116 123
https://www.samaritans.org/

**CALM (Campaign Against Living Miserably)**
Men's mental health and suicide prevention
5pm–midnight helpline 0800 58 58 58
https://www.thecalmzone.net/

**YOUNG MINDS**
Children's mental health – tools and resources for supporting
young people and their parents/carers/teachers
Parents' helpline 0808 802 5544
https://www.youngminds.org.uk/

**BIPOLAR UK**
Supporting people living with bipolar disorder
https://www.bipolaruk.org/

**NIGHTLINE ASSOCIATION**
Student-run nightline services at universities across the UK
https://nightline.ac.uk/

**BEAT**
The UK's leading charity for those suffering with eating disorders
https://www.beateatingdisorders.org.uk/

**RETHINK MENTAL ILLNESS**
Leading provider of regional mental health services and support
groups
https://www.rethink.org/

**OCD ACTION**
The UK's largest OCD charity, delivering frontline services
Helpline 0300 636 5478
https://ocdaction.org.uk/